Online Health Science Education

Development & Implementation

Online Health Science Education

Development & Implementation

- **Nalini Jairath**, PhD, RN
  Dean, School of Nursing
  The Catholic University of America
  Washington, DC

- **Mary Etta Mills**, RN, ScD, CNAA, FAAN
  Professor and Associate Dean for Academic Affairs
  University of Maryland School of Nursing
  Baltimore, Maryland

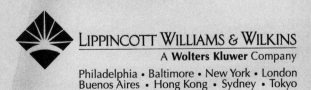

LIPPINCOTT WILLIAMS & WILKINS
A **Wolters Kluwer** Company

Philadelphia • Baltimore • New York • London
Buenos Aires • Hong Kong • Sydney • Tokyo

Senior Acquisitions Editor: Margaret Zuccarini
Managing Editor: Betsy Gentzler
Editorial Assistant: Marivette Torres
Production Project Manager: Cynthia Rudy
Director of Nursing Production: Helen Ewan
Senior Managing Editor / Production: Erika Kors
Art Director: Joan Wendt
Senior Manufacturing Manager: William Alberti
Production Services / Compositor: Schawk, Inc.
Printer: Donnelley–Crawfordsville

9 8 7 6 5 4 3 2 1

Library of Congress Cataloging-in-Publication Data

Online health science education : development and implementation / [edited by] Nalini Jairath,
Mary Etta Mills.— 1st ed.
    p. ; cm.
    Includes bibliographical references and index.
    ISBN 0-7817-5283-3 (alk. paper)
    1. Medicine—Study and teaching. 2. Paramedical education. 3. Distance education. I. Jairath, Nalini. II. Mills, Mary Etta C.
III. Title.
    [DNLM: 1. Health Personnel—education. 2. Education, Distance—methods. 3. Online Systems.
W 18 O585 2006]
R834.O65 2006
610′.7—dc22

                              2005022884

Care has been taken to confirm the accuracy of the information presented and to describe generally accepted practices. However, the authors, editors, and publisher are not responsible for errors or omissions or for any consequences from application of the information in this book and make no warranty, express or implied, with respect to the content of the publication.

The authors, editors, and publisher have exerted every effort to ensure that drug selection and dosage set forth in this text are in accordance with the current recommendations and practice at the time of publication. However, in view of ongoing research, changes in government regulations, and the constant flow of information relating to drug therapy and drug reactions, the reader is urged to check the package insert for each drug for any change in indications and dosage and for added warnings and precautions. This is particularly important when the recommended agent is a new or infrequently employed drug.

Some drugs and medical devices presented in this publication have Food and Drug Administration (FDA) clearance for limited use in restricted research settings. It is the responsibility of the health care provider to ascertain the FDA status of each drug or device planned for use in his or her clinical practice.

LWW.com

Dedication

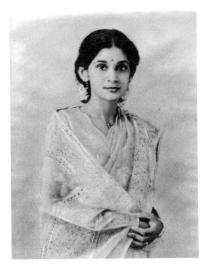

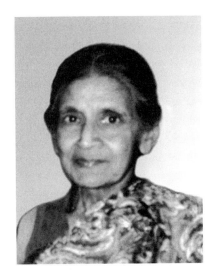

My mother, Juanita Jairath (1918–2001), lived a full and loving life despite many obstacles. Her intellectual challenge of the status quo and her persistence, faith, and optimism taught me, her conventional daughter, lessons that I am only beginning to appreciate following her death. This book is dedicated to my mother, as a celebration of her remarkable life.

Nalini Jairath

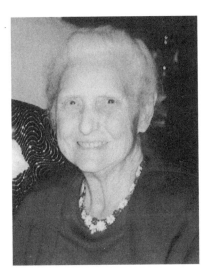

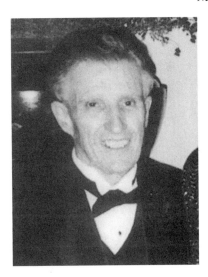

This book is dedicated to my mother, Mrs. Mary Jennings Mills, and my brother, Mr. Donald W. Mills, who supported me with their patience, understanding, and encouragement throughout years of working with the development and implementation of the online education programs and research that made this book possible.

Mary Etta Mills

Contributors

Barbara G. Covington, PhD, RN
Associate Dean for Information and Learning
    Technologies
Associate Professor, Organizational Systems
    and Adult Health
University of Maryland School of Nursing
Baltimore, Maryland

Shelley Jordon, BS
Multi-Media Technician, ITL
University of Maryland School of Nursing
Baltimore, Maryland

Michael Maranda, PhD
Evaluation Researcher
University of Maryland School of Nursing
Baltimore, Maryland

Dorothea McDowell, PhD, RN
Faculty/Associate Chair of Nursing
Henson School of Science & Technology
Salisbury University
Salisbury, Maryland

Ann Mech, JD, RN
Coordinator, Legal and Contractual Services
Associate Professor, Organizational Systems
    and Adult Health
University of Maryland School of Nursing
Baltimore, Maryland

Lyn Stankiewicz Murphy, MS, MBA, RN
Clinical Instructor
University of Maryland School of Nursing
Baltimore, Maryland

Savithramma Sanjoy, MS
Instructional Technology Specialist
University of Maryland School of Medicine
Baltimore, Maryland

Deborah Shpritz, PhD, RN
Program Director, Palliative Care Education
Adjunct Faculty, Johns Hopkins University
    School of Nursing
University of Maryland School of Medicine
Baltimore, Maryland

Debra L. Spunt, MS, RN
Clinical Instructor, Organizational Systems
Adult Health Director, Clinical Simulation
University of Maryland School of Nursing
Baltimore, Maryland

Nola Stair, MBA
Senior Information Technology Specialist
Center for Educational Resources (CER)
Johns Hopkins University
Baltimore, Maryland

Reviewers

Wanda Bonnel, PhD, RN
Clinical Associate Professor
University of Kansas
Kansas City, Kansas

JoEllen Datillo, PhD, RN
Assistant Dean for the Undergraduate Program
Georgia Baptist College of Nursing of Mercer
   University
Atlanta, Georgia

Denise R. Doliviera, MSN, RN
Associate Professor
Community College of Allegheny County,
   Boyce Campus
Monroeville, Pennsylvania

Betty Elder, MS, MSN
Assistant Professor
Wichita State University
Wichita, Kansas

Linda Foley, PhD, MSN, RN
Professor and Associate Chairperson, Curriculum
Nebraska Methodist College
Omaha, Nebraska

Ann M. Gothler, PhD, RN
Professor of Nursing
The Sage Colleges
Troy, New York

Paul J. Kapsar, MSN, RN, CRNP
Instructor
University of Pittsburgh School of Nursing
Pittsburgh, Pennsylvania

Cecilia Jane Maier, MS, RN, CCRN
Assistant Professor
Mount Carmel College of Nursing
Columbus, Ohio

Kimberly Hall Oas, MSN, RN, FNP-C
Instructor
Kent State University, College of Nursing
Kent, Ohio

May E. Phillips, PhD, RN
Consultant/Internet Faculty
Excelsior College and St. Joseph's College
Gettysburg, Pennsylvania

Kerry Risco, MSN, CRNP
Assistant Professor of Nursing
Slippery Rock University
Slippery Rock, Pennsylvania

Shari Stoops, MSN, RNC, FNC-P
Assistant Professor
Del Mar College
Corpus Christi, Texas

Joan Thiele, PhD, RN
Professor Emeritus
Washington State University
Spokane, Washington

Marleen Thornton, MSN, RN
Assistant Professor of Nursing
Alverno College
Milwaukee, Wisconsin

Preface

The past decade has seen an exponential increase in online education in the health sciences. Online education has been presented as a viable alternative to courses delivered using face-to-face methods, self-study, and other methods of distance education. Various educational benefits of online education as an emerging form of distance education have been cited, including the flexibility to accommodate students' diverse learning styles and schedules. As more institutions and academic programs join the online bandwagon, faculty are frequently given major responsibility for concurrently learning about and developing online programs and/or courses. Technological support and resources may be limited and faculty mentors nonexistent. The rapid, or in some cases immediate, learning curve faced by faculty can cause stress and affect their satisfaction with the faculty role. What should be an exciting opportunity to develop new teaching skills becomes a difficult process in which students and the quality of education may suffer.

As both academic administrators and faculty, we have seen the clear benefits of online education for preparing students in the health sciences for various professional roles. We have also encountered the same challenges faced by faculty as they seek to rapidly learn how to implement online courses and programs. There are relatively few resources beyond those provided by the companies that develop online courseware. The relevant research is limited, and published articles are replete with anecdotal information.

Online Health Science Education: Development & Implementation is targeted to the needs of health science faculty and to students taking coursework to prepare for clinical educator and faculty roles; it systematically addresses the development, implementation and evaluation of online courses, programs, and other educational offerings. Our hope is that this book will help faculty and future faculty enjoy their role in developing online courses and programs and appreciate the true potential of online education.

Organization

This book comprehensively explores the process of creating, offering, supporting, and evaluating online or web-based education. The content is organized around a web framework that shows the interrelationship of course-specific technological considerations, technologic components of the institutional infrastructure, legal and ethical considerations, and curricular components at the course level and at the academic program level. Details related to structural requirements, prerequisites, processes, and procedures required for functionality of desired outcomes and evaluation are presented in relation to the framework. Although the book is most effective when read in its entirety, we have structured each chapter to be of value when read in isolation.

The book is divided into four sections, beginning with a thorough discussion of infrastructure and program development. Based on the organizing web framework, an assessment method to determine the administrative, support, and fiscal requirements needed to develop and sustain web-based education in an academic environment is presented. Technical requirements and considerations necessary to online education are fully discussed, including legal considerations such as U.S. copyright law, elements of fair use, and the TEACH Act. Although we have used our experiences in the United States for illustration, similar issues are arising in other countries as online nursing education becomes globalized.

Section Two details the development of a virtual learning community, beginning with the method by which a solid needs assessment of student support requirements can be conducted and strategies developed to address gaps. Elements important to the implementation of online courses are discussed, including faculty selection factors, a systems approach to supporting faculty, and creation of decision rules underpinning online education.

Section Three addresses curricular considerations. Specific pedagogic models for online education are discussed, and model planning and evaluation of a curriculum to achieve learning outcomes are considered. The design, development, and implementation of individual courses are addressed in depth, from the selection of teaching approaches to the design of learning resources, incorporation of various communication venues, evaluation of instructors' performance, and achievement of learner outcomes.

In Section Four, special topics of increasing importance to online education are addressed. Evaluation of online courses is critical to the continual improvement of offerings. Methods are offered for instrument construction, design considerations, and analysis using the principle of triangulation. An innovative spectrum of clinical simulation for skill development and active learning in credit-bearing academic courses is presented. The use of strategic planning, design principles, and development considerations for online continuing education course development is detailed.

Approach

Because of the rapid rate of change in online education, *Online Health Science Education* emphasizes principles and practices that are responsive to changes in technology and courseware. The content builds on a base of experience, research, and knowledge. Our approach presents techniques shown to be successful in the planning, development, implementation, and evaluation of online education at the institutional planning and assessment level and at the individual course level. The book is based upon the premise that building a solid technical and administrative infrastructure, pedagogic model, and curriculum design are critical before creating and offering individual courses. Furthermore, we believe that an online enterprise, including individual course offerings, must be designed not only to meet student needs but also to provide faculty support through direct instructional design assistance and reasoned academic policies.

Special Features

The accessibility and usefulness of this book are enhanced by identification of learner objectives at the beginning of each chapter. Definitions of key terms also precede the chapter content, so that the reader will be better prepared to apply the terms in the intended context. Practical examples are included throughout the book to illustrate the application of content, and research is integrated throughout the chapters. At the end of each chapter, learning activities facilitate and challenge the reader in mastering the skills necessary to support the application of concepts and strategies offered in the book. A reference list offers sources for further reading on each subject. In line with the focus of this book, web citations as well as traditional journal and book citations are included.

This book is comprehensive in its content and provides a means for the reader to discover new knowledge or enhance current knowledge and skills in developing and implementing online health science education.

Nalini Jairath, PhD, RN
Mary Etta Mills, RN, ScD, CNAA, FAAN

Acknowledgments

We are grateful to the many faculty, staff, administrators, and students who have participated in the development, offering, support, and practical feedback of online courses and programs, which allowed us to provide practice and evidence-based content. Our special thanks go to the talented contributors who provided their knowledge and expertise for the benefit of health science educators immersed in the creation of innovative educational offerings. We also appreciate the efforts of the reviewers who contributed their time to critique the manuscript and offer suggestions for refinement. Our colleagues at the University of Maryland School of Nursing and throughout the United States have provided enthusiasm, scholarship, and professionalism as we have continually addressed issues in online education.

Contents

SECTION THREE

Curricular Considerations 103

SECTION FOUR

Special Topics 141

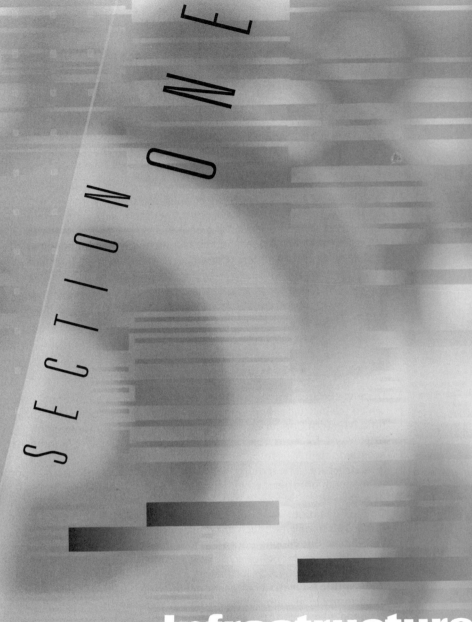

SECTION ONE

Infrastructure and Program Development

Objectives

Upon completion of this chapter, the learner will be able to:

- Define online education.
- Categorize the different types of online educational offerings.
- Identify the factors that have contributed to the growth of online education.
- Describe the components of a general framework for online education.
- Discuss the challenges faced by faculty involved with online education.
- Define new terms in this chapter.

Key Terms

Distance Education: A generic term that describes educational offerings in which the instructor and students are separated by location and potentially by time (Western Cooperative for Educational Telecommunication, http://www.wcet.info/resources/publications/conguide/conguida.htm, last accession date, December 2, 2003).

Infrastructure: The required facilities, services, and resources supporting educational programs within an academic institution or subunit (i.e., school, department).

Online Education: A type of distance education that uses the Internet/World Wide Web to deliver educational offerings to students.

Web-based Education: Education that uses the Internet/World Wide Web as the mechanism for delivery of course content and interactions between learners and teachers or facilitators.

Web-centric Education: Educational offerings in which web-based learning is the primary focus and delivery method; web-centric education is intermediate between web-based and web-enhanced education.

Web-enhanced Education: Education in which the Internet/World Wide Web is used to enhance or augment traditional educational approaches.

Web Presence: Education in which the Internet/World Wide Web is used selectively and in a limited way.

CHAPTER ONE

Overview of
Online Education

■ NALINI JAIRATH

Chapter Outline

W ithin the past decade, online education has been advocated as an innovative and practical approach for individuals preparing for careers in the health sciences or seeking advanced academic preparation. Online courses have been used successfully in a variety of ways across the various health disciplines. Therefore, knowledge and skills in the development, implementation, and evaluation of online offerings are beneficial to faculty and students preparing for clinical educator or faculty roles. Because of the rapid rate of change in online education, this book emphasizes content that goes beyond the limits of existing technology and current courseware.

This chapter provides a brief overview of online education and a framework for the development, implementation, and evaluation of online education in the health sciences. Subsequent chapters provide a more detailed exploration of specific aspects of online education.

ONLINE EDUCATION

Online education is a generic term that refers to the use of the Internet or World Wide Web (web) to deliver educational offerings to students (Jackson, 2001). Other related terms include e-learning, web education, and online distance education or distributive learning. Online education may encompass individual components of a course, individual courses, academic programs, and continuing educational offerings. The degree to which education is provided using online resources may vary, from courses that merely have a web presence to those that are completely web-based. Figure 1.1 presents the distinctions between the various types of online courses and programs and is based on common descriptions in the online literature. As indicated in this figure, online education need not be an all-or-nothing phenomenon; rather, it reflects the nature of the learning environment and the available learning resources.

THE CONTEXT OF ONLINE EDUCATION

Online education is an increasingly attractive educational option to both academic institutions and the student population. The number of online courses and online academic programs has grown exponentially within the United States and throughout the world. Although the actual benefit of online education continues to be evaluated, the growth has been fueled by trends affecting student enrollment, faculty attitudes and behaviors, academic expectations, technology, economics, and distance learning (Abromitis, 2002; Howell, Williams, & Lindsay, 2003). Some factors reflective of these trends are discussed in the following sections.

Minimizes Geographic Barriers

First, online education has the potential to increase an academic institution's pool of prospective students by minimizing geographic barriers to course or program attendance. Traditionally, the academic mission of educational institutions relates to the needs of a

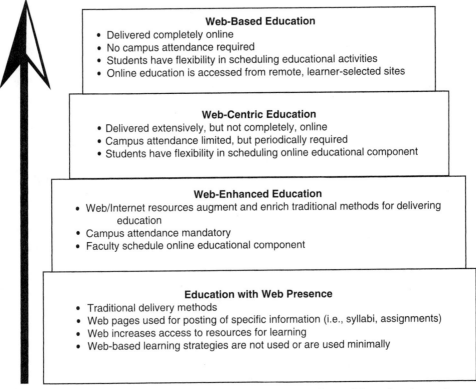

FIGURE 1.1 Types of online education based on the degree of use of the web or Internet.

geographically defined student population. Students are recruited from geographically discrete areas and are required to do coursework on campus or to participate in distance education through transmission to remote sites.

Eliminates Lifestyle Barriers

Second, online education eliminates educational barriers related to lifestyle constraints that make regular, on-site attendance at campus-based sessions difficult or undesirable. Shift workers, administrators, individuals whose work requires travel, and those whose family commitments make regular attendance in traditional programs difficult have greater opportunities through online education. The nature of many health science careers requires shift work and regular schedule changes. Therefore, online education is a practical solution to the challenges faced by students in health science careers (Kenner, Androwich, & Edwards, 2003).

Responds to Learning Style Needs of Adults

Third, online education is conceptualized and implemented using approaches that are respectful and responsive to the learning styles and learning needs of adult learners

(Hutchins, 2003). Because of differences in entry-level requirements for practice as well as work history for students pursuing advanced education in their field, flexibility in the content and depth of educational offerings is important. Effective online education focuses on the recipients as active, self-directed learners whose interest and educational gaps in particular topics may vary widely. In online education, the teacher is a *facilitator* who provides learners with opportunities to individualize their learning, tailor it to their unique circumstances, and use multiple, complementary methods to meet learning objectives.

Is Economically Feasible

Finally, online education is increasingly feasible to implement with technological advances that lower the cost, increase the speed of access, and enhance the quality of transmitted information. Online education also eliminates or reduces costs associated with student relocation to be close to the geographic campus and the need to scale back the number of hours of employment because of conflicts between work hours and the time courses or programs are offered.

A FRAMEWORK FOR ONLINE EDUCATION

All educational offerings require a supportive infrastructure. In traditional education where academic programs are well-established, faculty may have limited involvement in the development, maintenance, and enhancement of this infrastructure. In contrast, in online education the process of infrastructure development may not be clearly understood or articulated. Although enthusiasm for online education may be high among administrators and students, the necessary expertise may not be available. In these circumstances, faculty play a pivotal role in infrastructure design and may have to troubleshoot when infrastructure issues impact the quality of online education.

In Section One of this book, a framework is presented to help readers understand the infrastructure for development, implementation, and evaluation of online education; the framework is based on earlier work (Jairath & Stair, 2004). It is congruent with existing analyses, guidelines, recommendations, and policies regarding instructional technology, web pedagogical literature, and traditional approaches to curriculum design and reflects lessons learned in developing, implementing, and evaluating web-based courses in the School of Nursing at the University of Maryland–Baltimore.

Online education may be understood in terms of three major components: (a) technological, (b) legal and administrative, and (c) curricular (Figure 1.2). Each component may be further understood as having elements that are specific to certain types of courses and those pertinent to the entire range of online offerings. The relative importance and nature of the infrastructure issues may differ during the development, implementation, and evaluation phases. Potential and actual problems may be minimized when infrastructure developers and stakeholders address structural requirements or prerequisites, processes and procedures required for functionality, and desired outcomes.

Nursing Web Framework

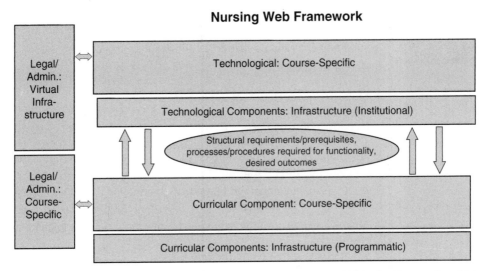

FIGURE 1.2 Nursing web framework. First published in *Nursing Education Perspectives*, Vol. 25, No. 2, March/April 2004, p. 68. Used with permission of Dr. Nalini N. Jairath.

Technological Components

The technological components are those specifically required for the development, delivery, and sustainability of online education. The technological component encompasses equipment, technological resources, and support services required for effective functioning. Although course-specific technological requirements exist, the larger infrastructure supporting the web-based course is particularly important because it provides the context for online education at a particular institution. Box 1.1 summarizes criteria for the technological infrastructure. These criteria are based on our experience and are congruent with "Quality on the Line: Benchmarks for Success in Internet-based Distance Education" (Institute for Higher Education Policy, 2000).

Capabilities of Available Resources and Resultant Outcomes

As noted in Box 1.1, available resources must be congruent with the desired outcomes of online education. These resources, which include equipment and access to support personnel, will be discussed in great detail in subsequent chapters. In general, inadequate technology may impose time delays or lags in transmission of information between the remote and on-campus sites. This may constrain communication between students, faculty, and on-site classmates. In addition, if transmission to the remote site is impaired due to technological difficulties, students at the remote site may be disadvantaged through missed classes or classes of poor quality. All of these issues may affect the quality of learning experienced by students enrolled in distance education. In contrast, when properly implemented, online education facilitates equal treatment of students by eliminating distance-based differences in the quality of teaching and the quality of communication within the class.

Criteria for Technological Infrastructure Component

BOX 1.1

Capabilities of available resources and resultant outcomes:

- Server hardware
- Courseware packages
- Multimedia development tools
- Graphic design software
- Network connectivity
- Troubleshooting procedures
- Technical and instructional design support personnel to consistently meet anticipated student utilization

Ongoing associated costs of upgrading to enhance the technological performance of server capacity and network connectivity:

- Processes to ensure the existence of minimum technological expertise and resources
- Computer hardware and peripherals
- Software
- Institutional e-mail accounts
- Internet access
- Modem speed necessary for students to participate in a web-based course

Flexibility and Feasibility of Upgrading

In addition to having a currently adequate infrastructure, viable high-quality systems must be flexible and permit expansion as consumer demand for online education increases and as the resources available via the Internet increase in scope and complexity. Because the lifetime of specific equipment is limited and upgrades to existing equipment occur relatively frequently and may be associated with significant improvements in quality and performance, a crucial objective during infrastructure development is to ensure that the structural features, processes, and procedures are adaptable, responsive, and upgradable in an efficient and cost-effective manner.

The technological infrastructure must also be flexible enough to facilitate easy access and usage of course materials from a variety of Internet-connected environments. Currently, these environments may use personal computer (PC) or cable modems, digital subscriber lines (DSL), local area networks with dedicated T-1 lines, and, to an increasing degree, wireless and satellite technology. An inflexible or inadequately responsive infrastructure may ultimately limit student access to information and necessitate modification of the methods used to deliver course content. Because each institution's environment and usage requirements vary, infrastructure requirements may differ across institutional settings.

Course-Specific Technological Requirements

The technological infrastructure must support the requirements for specific courses, as summarized in Box 1.2. Our experience indicates that health sciences courses with clinical, laboratory, or health informatics components pose unique challenges and provide the

Criteria for Course-Specific Technological Component

Need for plug-ins and additional equipment:
- PC digital video (i.e., eyeball) cameras
- Video and audio players and software

Relationship between students' ability to perform course-specific computations and required calculations:
- Processing speeds
- Modem capabilities
- PC memory requirements

opportunity for creative online solutions. With clinical courses, hands-on patient care is frequently a requisite component. Similarly, frequent faculty feedback and evaluation of student performance in the clinical setting is mandatory for patient safety and for student learning. These mandates can be addressed in the online environment through development of alternate arrangements for faculty to evaluate student performance. For example, eyeball cameras connected to laptop computers when students are in the clinical setting or the use of standardized patients for performance evaluation represent potentially viable alternatives. Similarly, although aspects of the laboratory setting may be duplicated in a virtual environment, the additional knowledge gained from direct performance of laboratory experiments may be difficult to duplicate. The process of cadaver dissection illustrates the challenges and potential solutions on online education. Online, three-dimensional cross sections of tissues and organ systems may be magnified, transformed to illustrate the impact of specific diseases on anatomical structure, and rotated to present images that are hidden because of cadaveric position.

Legal and Administrative Components

This section addresses the infrastructure required to manage and develop online education in accord with legal requirements and sound administrative practice. These two factors are inextricably linked with legal factors driving some aspects of the administrative structure of a program. For example, legal requirements may dictate the way in which course grades and program records may be stored electronically. As with the technology component, course-specific legal and administrative requirements are subsumed under the general legal and administrative components of the online educational infrastructure. The required legal and administrative or virtual infrastructure depends on the scope and nature of the program through which online education is offered. For web-based courses offered as part of continuing education, the virtual infrastructure requirements may be limited in that the registration process is relatively simple and a large array of student support services related to student progression through an academic program may not be necessary. However, for online courses taken as part of degree, diploma, or certificate programs, infrastructure requirements are more complex with respect to record keeping, monitoring of student compliance with health record requirements, malpractice requirements, and provision of academic counseling. Although similar to those requirements for supporting other courses or academic programs, the virtual infrastructure should be explicitly structured to eliminate on-campus attendance. Mills, Fisher, and Stair (2001) recommend that the virtual infrastructure approximate the campus-based services and facilities related to registration and records, financial aid, student orientation, academic advisement, counseling, library resources, support services, writing centers, student appeals, evaluation, and assessment. Box 1.3 indicates the criteria for the legal and administrative components that will be addressed in great detail in subsequent chapters. As noted in this box, much of the legal and administrative structure pertains to developing processes and mechanisms to ensure compliance with legal requirements and efficient student transitions through the online program.

Course-Specific Legal and Administrative Requirements

As with traditional courses, the administrative structure of web-based courses and resultant expectations of students should be clearly articulated. Our experience

Criteria for Legal and Administrative Infrastructure Component

BOX 1.3

Articulation approaches between:

- Course software
- Student registration
- Student tracking and monitoring approaches

Mechanisms for the student:

- Face-to-face or web-based orientation
- Support for online education
- Communication

Development of administrative mechanisms to facilitate student access to teaching materials

Development of online student handbook(s) delineating expectations for performance in web-based courses or web-based academic programs

Policies to address the impact of web-based teaching on faculty workload

Administrative approaches to ensure the integrity of online exams or to establish proctoring arrangements when exams cannot be administered online

Increased legal access by students to copyrighted or protected material through:

- Site licensing arrangements
- Shareware and freeware programs
- Public domain web resources
- Library accessible electronic reserve systems
- Remote access library services with gateways to electronic copies of health science journals

suggests that some students may confuse the adaptability of online courses to their learning needs with a relatively archaic, completely student-directed approach to course participation and completion of course assignments. For example, students may opt to complete all their assignments at the beginning of a semester or do the majority of work within a few specific weeks. If the course material requires time for integration, learning may be impaired. Box 1.4 identifies criteria for the legal and administrative component of specific courses. These criteria were identified based on the online educational literature and the author's experiences with web education. Many of the criteria deal with acceptable use by students of online resources and student recognition of the legal issues associated with privacy of communications (cyber security). Others deal with the translation of traditional learning venues and approaches into online venues and approaches.

Criteria for Legal and Administrative Course-Specific Component

BOX 1.4

Faculty's minimal expectations of student accountability for periodic communication through:

- E-mails
- Synchronous and asynchronous communications
- Participation in group work
- Acceptable and respectful online behaviors

Acceptable use of online communication venues:

- Group chat rooms
- Course and group home pages
- Synchronous and asynchronous discussion areas

Limits to confidentiality and privacy of e-mails and postings in these communication venues

Procedures and accommodations for hardware or connectivity issues that limit ability to access and participate in the course:

- Computer viruses
- Malfunctioning computers

Procedures for completing, submitting, maintaining security, and addressing security breaches of online assignments, exams, and other forms of evaluation

Maintaining consistency and equivalence between web-based and traditional sections of multisection courses with respect to:

- Course content
- Sequencing of course material
- Evaluation approaches
- Student course-related expenditures for books, supplies, and learning resources

Curricular Component

The curricular component of the online educational infrastructure must permit attainment of the terminal and intermediate objectives of educational programs and be compatible with the teaching and learning approaches, or pedagogy, that guide the educational program (Barton, 1997). Unlike the technological, legal, and administrative components, there is no clear delineation between course-specific and general curricular components. Considerable debate exists regarding the philosophical approach that should guide curricula involving the use of online learning. For adult learners such as those in health science programs, constructivist approaches (Brown, 2000; Cole, 2000; Reeves, 1997) that emphasize active learning, student self-direction, and the use of multiple resources and learning modalities have been advocated for inclusion in online education. However, to accommodate potential variations in learning styles of online learners and time limitations in many health science programs, a purely constructivist approach may not be helpful. Additional information about the various pedagogical approaches is found in subsequent chapters.

From a curricular perspective, regardless of the pedagogical approach that dominates particular online educational offerings, web-based courses also differ from traditional courses in terms of the teaching approaches used and, possibly, the evaluative approaches. Simple transference of traditional teaching approaches may not capitalize on the inherent flexibility and opportunity associated with web-based education. Box 1.5 identifies specific criteria for the curricular component. These pertain to the way in which learning occurs in online programs and courses. Once again, this component and these criteria will be addressed in greater detail in subsequent chapters. Our experience suggests that certain methods, such as the use of guest speakers, are relatively easy because presentations can be taped beforehand and then used as necessary. However, content that requires in-class practice or detailed coaching by faculty may require the development of web-based tutorials, the use of technology, such as eyeball cameras to transmit visual information back to faculty, or the use of multiple, complementary methods of learning. Our experience suggests that, at the undergraduate level, texts should be selected that are detailed, comprehensive, and easy to read. Additional teaching approaches are used to highlight or explore content in greater detail, but it may be helpful for faculty to recognize that some students may opt to skip content presented using other formats. Students may opt out because of technical difficulties with accessing additional resources. Students whose orientation focuses on mastery of content required for exams may also view the additional resources as supplemental and too costly in terms of their time commitment.

Criteria for Program and Course-Specific Curricular Components

BOX 1.5

- Curricular focus of content or method selected
- Feasibility of developing teaching and learning approaches
- Visual and auditory appeal
- Complexity of course material
- Adaptability to learner needs and their needs for upgrading of materials

CONCLUSION

In this chapter, a brief introduction to and an infrastructure for the development and evaluation of online education have been presented. When the technological, legal and administrative, and curricular components of the infrastructure are carefully addressed, online education in the health sciences can potentially enhance student learning, progression through educational programs, and satisfaction with the educational experience.

■ LEARNING ACTIVITIES

● Conduct a web search to determine the commonalities and differences between the ways in which the terms *e-learning*, *online learning*, *distance education*, and *distributive education* are used.

● Go to the Distance Education Clearinghouse web site at http://www.uwex.edu/disted. Examine the definitions of distance learning. In addition to online education, what are the other types of distance learning?

● Review the Institute for Higher Education Policy's landmark position paper "Quality on the Line: Benchmarks for Success in Internet-based Distance Education." This paper may be found by following the publication links at www.ihep.com. Identify and discuss the five criteria related to faculty support for online education.

● Go to the web site for the *Online Journal of Distance Learning Administration* at http://www.westga.edu/~distance/jmain11.html. Review the following article: "Thirty two trends affecting distance education: An informed foundation for strategic planning" (Howell, William, & Lindsay, 2003). Of the 32 identified trends, select the five most important trends affecting the development of online education within your profession.

● Go to the web site for the *Electronic Journal of e-learning* at www.ejel.org. Review the following article: "Biomedical online learning: The route to success" (Harvey, Cookson, Meerabeau, & Muggleston, 2003). Compare the framework presented for online courses with Figure 1.2. Discuss the relative merits of the two frameworks and their compatibility with each other.

REFERENCES

Abromitis, J. (2002). Trends in instructional technology and distance education. (ERIC Document Reproduction Service No. ED472650). Retrieved August 26, 2005, from http://www.eric.ed.gov.

Barton, K. (1997). Constructivism vs. instructivism. Retrieved August 26, 2005, from University of South Carolina, College of Education web site: http://www.ed.sc.edu/caw/webbarton.htm

Brown, D. G. (Ed.) (2000). *Interactive learning.* (2nd ed.) Bolton, MA: Anker Publishing.

Cole, R. (Ed.) (2000). *Issues in web-based pedagogy: A critical primer.* Westport, CT: Greenwood.

Harvey, P. J., Cookson, B., Meerabeau, E., & Muggleston, D. (2003). Biomedical online learning: The route to success on behalf of the Steering Committee of the Biomedical Online Learning Project. *Electronic Journal of e-learning, 1*(1), Article number. Retrieved December 3, 2003, from http://www.ejel.org/issue-1/issue1-art4.htm

Howell, S. L., Williams P. B., & Lindsay N. K. (2003). Thirty two trends affecting distance education: An informed foundation for strategic planning. *Online Journal of Distance Learning Administration, 6*(3). Retrieved August 26, 2005, from http://www.westga.edu/~distance/ojdla/fall63/howell63.html

Hutchins, H. M. (2003). Instructional immediacy and the seven principles: Strategies for facilitating online courses. *Online Journal of Distance Learning Administration, 6*(3). Retrieved December 3, 2003, from http://www.westga.edu/~distance/ojdla/fall63/hutchins63.html

The Institute for Higher Education Policy. (2000). Quality on the line: Benchmarks for success in Internet-based distance education. Retrieved August 26, 2005, from http://www.ihep.com/Pubs/PDF/Quality.pdf

Jackson, R. H. (2001). Web based learning resources library—A bibliography of web based educational tools, theory and practices. Retrieved August 26, 2005, from http://www.knowledgeability.biz/weblearning/

Jairath, N., & Stair, N. (2004). A development and implementation framework for Web-based nursing courses. *Nursing Education Perspectives, 25*(2), 67–72.

Kenner, C., Androwich, I. M., & Edwards, P. A. (2003). Innovative educational strategies to prepare nurse executives for new leadership roles. *Nursing Administration Quarterly, 27*(2), 172–179.

Mills, M. E., Fisher, C., & Stair, N. (2001). Web-based courses: More than curriculum. *Nursing & Health Care Perspectives, 22*(5), 235–239.

Reeves, T. (1997). Evaluating what really matters in computer-based education. Retrieved August 26, 2005, from http://www.educationau.edu.au/archives/cp/REFS/reeves.htm

Western Cooperative for Educational Telecomunications. (1999). The distance learner's guide. Retrieved August 26, 2005, from http://cwx.prenhall.com/dlguide

Objectives

Upon completion of this chapter, the learner will be able to:

- Discuss the elements necessary for the development and sustainability of a web-based program.
- Design and analyze an infrastructure needs assessment necessary to develop and sustain a web-based educational program in an academic environment.
- Formulate administrative and support requirements, as well as other essential components necessary to develop and sustain web-based education in an academic environment.
- Create and critically evaluate an appropriate costing model for an academic web-based program, including infrastructure development and sustainment.

Key Terms

Benefit–Cost Ratio (BCR): Also known as profitability index; compares the number of dollars of benefit to each dollar of cost.

Break-Even Analysis (BEA): An analytical technique that helps determine the level of volume needed to reach the financial break-even point of an investment.

Institutional Supports: The resources and technical support that must be dedicated to the program or course offering.

Return on Investment (ROI): A financial ratio (earnings divided by investments); examines the percentage gain or loss experienced from an investment; used to compare opportunities inside or outside an organization.

Scale of the Offering: The size or largeness of program or course offering.

Scope of the Offering: The dimensions of the program or course offering while satisfying a given set of specified conditions.

CHAPTER TWO

Administrative Infrastructure

■ BARBARA G. COVINGTON AND
LYN STANKIEWICZ MURPHY

Chapter Outline

his chapter will provide course developers, program developers, educators, administrative personnel, learners, and others an overview of the needs assessment, administrative, and support requirements, as well as the essential keys necessary to develop, sustain, and evaluate a web-based education program in an academic environment. It will focus on information that is applicable across a wide variety of settings and types of programs. After completing this chapter, the reader will be able to selectively identify issues, decide on alternatives, and answer questions that are unique to his or her situation.

Education today is no longer limited to the traditional physical classroom to which most of us are accustomed. Education can now be delivered via the World Wide Web, where learners can be exposed to education from just about any setting or environment, whether it is at home, in an office, or in an Internet cafe. Although the interaction between instructors and learners in online education may seem different from the traditional physical classroom education in its delivery and options, the communication between the two remain unchanged. Simonson, Smaldino, Albright, and Zvacek (2003) describe communication as the interaction between two individuals in order to share ideas. Communication in the traditional classroom and online education occurs when learners interact with one another and with the instructor. The only difference is that in online education, the communication or the ability to convey information, is delivered via technology. This method of delivery, as well as the nature of web-based courses and programs, varies based on a number of factors, such as cost, technological support, and other resources.

DELIVERY OF ONLINE EDUCATION

Delivery methods of online education usually range from audio, two-way video, web-enhanced or hybrid course, to web-based or webcentric course. An audio program may consist of an audiotaping of a lecture to which the learner will listen. Visual supplements, such as PowerPoint slides, may accompany the audio lecture, but the audio program provides a voice-only connection between the learner and the instructor. This type of audiotaping was quite popular for a number of years; however, its main use today is for self-help materials for individual study (Simonson, et al., 2003). Similarly, video learning is comparable to that of audio, with the learner viewing a video clip or video stream of the instructor, rather than listening to an audio recording. The barrier for both of these two types of online education delivery is that there is only a one-way communication stream: instructor to learner. To enhance the communication between the learner and the instructor, two-way video or video conferencing may be used. This type of delivery method consists of live video and audio communication from two or more locations. The advantage to this type of online education is that the learner and instructor can interact and experience two-way communication. A web-enhanced, or hybrid course, "is one in which some face-to-face learning experiences are replaced by virtual learning experiences or technology enhanced strategies" (O'Neil, Fisher, & Newbold, 2004, p. 1). Thus, web-enhanced education maintains the traditional principles of a physical classroom education, while weaving throughout aspects of web-based instruction. Lastly, web-based or web-centric education is education or training that is delivered over the Internet and accessible using a browser. Web-based education is known as anytime, anywhere learning; it is asynchronous learning, learning that takes place over the Internet without everyone being present at the same time, or delayed learning (O'Neil, et al., 2004).

In order to be successful in any of these types of online education courses or programs, the appropriate infrastructure for the web-based program must be addressed and readily understood by the users of the program. Regardless if one is in the middle of an established online educational program or about to start the planning and implementation for one, taking the time to methodically consider and plan for infrastructure requirements and program development will be beneficial in the long run for all users involved. These efforts will assist in assessing the strengths and weaknesses of the program, as well as improve the chances of producing and maintaining a successful program in a healthy form.

SCOPE, SCALE, AND SUPPORT OF EDUCATIONAL OFFERINGS

For any partial or fully online education program to exist in a healthy form, careful attention has to be paid to three areas:

1. The scope of the offering.
2. The scale of the offering.
3. The institutional supports of the offering.

Scope of the offering refers to the dimensions of the program or course offering while satisfying a given set of specified conditions. In understanding the scope, one is able to establish the goals and objectives of the program from development, implementation, and evaluation, as well as the environment in which the program exists. No matter how carefully a program is planned, it is almost certain that the scope will change before completion. These changes may be related to error identification, technological advancements, an increase in education or sophistication, client/user mandate, or organizational demands. How one manages the scope of the program is critical to the success of the program.

Scale of the offering refers to the size of the program or course offering. By identifying the scale of the offering, one is able to identify the resources necessary to establish and sustain the program. For example, an organization may decide that based on scope, scale, and support, core classes of a specific academic program may be created as online, web-based education. However, in another organization, the goal of the organization is to have the entire academic program available as online or web-based education. Again, scale of the offering is dependent on the resources and support of the organization, as well as the scope of the organization.

Lastly, institutional supports refer to the resources and technical support that must be dedicated to the program or course offering (Meredith & Mantel, 2000). Support is again dependent on the organization and will assist in determining the scope and scale of the offerings.

Clearly, there exists unique linkages and dependency between these three entities of scope, scale, and institutional supports. The complexity, nature, and dependency of these linkages intensifies and weakens as course offerings move from a traditional delivery method of classroom teaching to a completely online course program. One prominent factor in the strength or weakness of the relationships is the stage of planning, implementation, or evaluation in which the user is engaged. For example, the scope of attention needed for the day-to-day operations (routine maintenance and short-term requirements) is equal to the scope of attention needed for the long-range ownership and maintenance of the infrastructure elements. However, the scale of the short-term offering may be smaller than the scale of the offering planned for the future. Thus, it is imperative for the organization to focus not only on the present, but on the future as well. Insufficient planning for the future is not healthy and can result in failure. Projecting a skeptical eye to the future may seem gloomy to some program developers, but it makes good sense (Meredith & Mantel, 2000). Thus, in order to achieve this, attention must be divided between the short-term, or operational, goals and objectives of the program, as well as the long-term, or strategic, goals and objectives of the program.

NEEDS ASSESSMENT OF EXISTING PROGRAMS: A NEW FOCUS

Because models of delivery vary based on the scope, scale, and support of the program offering, the focus of this chapter will be on an average program offering. In online education, much of the literature advocates that program guidelines and suggestions need to be educationally and economically sound, with the focus actually being the customers (learner and teacher) rather than the educational product itself. This shift away from the educational product (i.e., putting a course online) to the relationship between the learner and instructor may be a new idea for some. This new focus on the learner–educator dyad allows the program developer to develop (or refine) a program, starting at the planning stage, with the customer, both internal and external, in mind. Thus, the goal of the new focus is that the end product matches the needs of the user rather the organization that developed it. This approach allows the developer to examine the users, their changing needs and wants, and the response to those changes (Billings, 2000; Draves, 2002). This dynamic method shifts our focus from the present environment to the ever-present changing environment and allows for current and future programs to be customer-focused and customer-friendly while encompassing the appropriate content in order to meet the needs in terms of the short-term and long-term goals of the organization.

Cost

The first point of discussion for any program and/or infrastructure development is the overall cost of the project. This basic question of "What does it cost to create an online educational program?" is not easily answered. The literature reports that reasonable estimates for web-based courses and programs are reported in the range of $3,000 to over $250,000 for development and implementation (Bates, 2000; Bourne & Moore, 2001). However, a great deal of discrepancy exists in determining actual costs of web-based education offering or program in the literature. Bates (2000) stated that to find the underlying costs of web-based education, distinctive categories must be created. Costs that should be factored include: costs for infrastructure, equipment, and materials for the offering of the courses (capital costs); costs that occur on an ongoing basis, such as information technology support (recurrent costs); development or production costs; delivery costs; and fixed costs such as faculty development (Bartolic-Zlomislic & Bates, 1999; Bates, 2000). Of these costs, technology infrastructure is the "largest cost hurdle" (Morgan, 2005, p. 14). One point to keep in mind is that these costs reflect the development of the course offering. Additional costs, such as faculty and support personnel costs, must also be considered when teaching the course. Marshall University estimated that the cost of developing an online course was $301,330.80, while the cost of teaching the same course online was $225,568.63 (Morgan, 2005). Thus, organizations must be aware of planning for costs in both development and teaching phases of the course offering. The interesting point is that the literature has demonstrated that, in reality, there is a lack of consistency in costing and reporting methods for web-based programs. Thus, there is not one correct way or model to cost these types of offerings.

Traditionally three costing approaches have been used for analyzing most web-based programs: benefit–cost ratio (BCR), return on investment (ROI), and break-even analysis (BEA) (Phillips, 1994; Phillips, 2002; Whalen & Wright, 1999). Benefit–cost analysis (BCA), also known as profitability index, compares the number of dollars of benefit to each dollar of cost. In effect, it tells how many dollars are gained for each dollar invested. The benefit–cost ratio is the present value of total benefits divided by present value of total costs. The first step in conducting a BCA is to identify the components of the analysis: costs and benefits. Costs are the resources required as inputs and must be measurable in monetary units such as dollars. Costs may be classified as direct costs, that is, costs that are directly related to, or used as inputs in the production of an objective function, such as a web-based program. Examples of direct costs are the salaries of the staff, faculty, equipment, and so on. Additionally, indirect costs must be measured. Indirect costs are those costs that are not used directly toward the production of the web-based course, such as office space, lighting, heating, and other incidentals. Again, both costs and benefits must be expressed as tangible inputs that can be converted to monetary units such as dollars. Benefits are the outputs or contributions, produced by the objective function, the web-based program. For example, new knowledge of learners may be a benefit to web-based courses; convenience may be a benefit of a web-based program. Benefits must also be expressed in tangible outputs that can be converted to monetary units such as dollars, however, this is often difficult because many of the benefits of web-based education are intangible items such as gained knowledge.

Next, it is important to remember that both values of cost and benefits must be converted into present value using appropriate discounting methods. Discounting is converting the future value of monetary units into its present value. Discounting enables the calculation and analysis of costs and benefits for specified number of years into the future (Penner, 2004). Once these data are obtained, the BCA may be calculated. The BCA is calculated as follows: BC ratio = total benefits ÷ total costs. For example, if the total benefits for a web-based program is $425,000 and the total cost is $325,000, the BC ratio equals $425,000 ÷ $325,000 or 1.30. In other words, the web-based program generates $1.30 of benefits for every dollar of cost.

The second approach is return on investment (ROI), which examines the percentage gain or loss experienced from an investment. Organizations must produce returns on their investments greater than the cost of capital used to finance their investment. ROI increases as net income increases for fixed amounts of invested capital. In other words, the more income an organization earns with its invested capital, the better the ROI. It is important to remember that ROI is often meaningless for future decisions. An ROI based on historical costs tells you how well the investment has done, not how well it will do in the future. For example, a university could not borrow money at 10% and invest the proceeds in projected earnings of 6% and expect to stay in business (Cleverly & Cameron, 2003).

The third approach is break-even analysis (BEA). BEA is an analytical technique that helps determine the level of volume needed to reach the financial break-even point of an investment; that is, the point at which net revenue exactly equals cost. At this point, there is neither a loss nor a profit. Of special interest is the point at which the investment in a business opportunity will be profitable. Break-even analysis in this case determines the output volume at which the profits from the opportunity equals zero (Ward, 1994).

A break-even analysis relies on the decomposition of costs into fixed and variable costs. Fixed costs are those costs that are independent of the level of production or volume. Variable costs are those costs that change proportionally with the level of production or volume. They represent resources whose consumption can be adjusted to match the demand placed for them. A break-even chart can visually present alternative profits and losses based on volume. To illustrate, consider the following example. A university has the following financial data:

- Variable costs per web-based course: $1,000.
- Fixed costs per web-based course: $25,000.
- Price per web-based course per learner: $1,500.

The break-even analysis can be determined by dividing fixed costs by the contribution margin (the difference between price and variable costs). Thus, in our example, the break-even analysis would be $25,000 ÷ ($1,500 − $1,000) or 50 learners. If the university enrolls 50 or more learners, then the university will make a profit, but if the volume goes below 50 learners, the university will incur a loss in its web-based program.

Although these financial analyses provide a mathematical basis for the evaluation of the program, there are opportunities to miss influential and opportunity costs. This may occur for a number of reasons. These methods require information that may not be well defined or available to the program planner or developer. Because the stakeholders of web-based education and the objectives for delivering or planning to offer web-based education cover a broad spectrum where one method may be appropriate and another may not, it may be similar to trying to push a square peg into a round hole (Figure 2.1).

For example, a program offered in a for-profit environment may be assessed using ROI, whereas in a nonprofit environment, BCA may determine the value of the program. The issue then arises when comparing the programs in terms of two different types of analyses. Further complicating the choice of costing methods is that, in either type of program, some may be fully or partially subsidized by a grant or private or public funding and expected to show, at a minimum, a breakeven on money invested by the organiza-

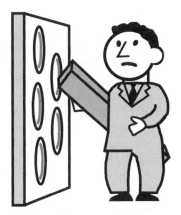

FIGURE 2.1 Fitting a square peg (program funding) into a round hole (program costs).

tion. In conclusion, the actual cost model settled on for planning and or monitoring the success of the program might be a combination of the above methods.

Commitment

In order for any new program, project, or course offering to be successful, it must be included as part of the organization's vision and mission statement, as well as the strategic plan. These components of the organization demonstrate the purpose of the organization (mission), where it sees itself in the future (vision), and the method by which these two entities will be achieved (strategic plan) (Daft, 1998). With regard to web-based education, the strategic plan is most important. The strategic plan defines the organization and acts as a framework for future decisions. From the strategic plan, an organization's mission statement is derived. The mission statement identifies the organization's constituency and specifically addresses its aim and function. The mission reflects how the organization plans to use its resources to gain a competitive advantage in the marketplace. The mission statement is the highest priority in the planning hierarchy as it influences the development of the organization's philosophy and goals, from which the objectives, policies, and procedures giving direction to the staff of the organization are derived (Marquis & Huston, 1994). It is the responsibility of management to ensure all employees are knowledgeable in the mission and strategic plan of an organization (i.e., get the word out). The purpose of having all employees aware of the mission and strategic plan is so all are working toward the same common goals and objectives—singing from the same song sheet. This can be achieved through posting the mission statement throughout an organization, providing copies for all employees, and holding assemblies or meetings to communicate this information. Often, individuals are employed in organizations where an individual's value or philosophy may differ from the philosophy or value of the organization. This may result in great personal conflict. The greatest safeguard against this type of conflict is for individuals to obtain a copy of the philosophy and/or mission statement of the organization prior to employment (Daft, 1998; Marquis & Huston, 1994).

The University of Maryland School of Nursing's Mission Statement and Web Education Direction Statement clearly demonstrate the commitment of the school's resources to the development of web-based education. From this, web-based education has a place of priority within the School of Nursing. It is important for all employees, both faculty and staff of the school, to be familiar with and accept the mission statement and have goals and objectives that coincide with that of the organization's mission for developing web-based education. Thus, it should not be a surprise to find that other traditional opportunities for learning may take a backseat to that of web-based education. It is critical to determine the existence of commitment within the organization. The wording may be specific or general in nature, but the presence of wording indicates that support of the program within the organization has begun. An example may be as follows: "...the organization as a leader in incorporating state-of-the-art technology to enhance the quality and efficiency of education that embraces the use of distance education across all levels of the curriculum and life-long continuing education activities." Or the wording may be to the effect that "it supports the use of web education as both an enhancement to traditional classes and for full web-based distance learning opportunities." Other examples may present as "a balance between web and traditional classroom approach to education to ensure the needs of the diverse learner population are met and the selection of the appropriate teaching strategy for our courses is completed."

If the commitment is not stated or present within the organization, it is essential that a statement be built in as soon as possible in the planning phase. Some points to consider may include additions to the mission statement, strategic plan, or 5-year plan. These commitments will allow administration flexibility and innovation support for at least some form of distance education. A formal process for project development with input from stakeholders is critical. In this case, the development team must include the customers (learners and teachers), and technical and administrative staff.

An example of the type of commitment needed is found in the December 2003 Direction Statement of the University of Maryland School of Nursing Ad Hoc Web Education Committee. The statement is as follows:

The University of Maryland School of Nursing, as a leader in incorporating state of the art technology to enhance the quality and efficiency of nursing education, embraces the use of web education across all levels of the curriculum and life long continuing education activities.

The School of Nursing supports the use of web education as both an enhancement to traditional classes and for full web-based distance learning opportunities. We believe a balance must be maintained between web and traditional classroom approach to education to insure we are meeting the needs of our diverse learner population and the selection of the appropriate teaching strategy for our courses.

In line with the school's mission, strategic plan, and the finite number of resources available, priorities will be assigned to new and existing projects. These priorities will assist in workload management and resources allocation decisions. When appropriate and possible, outside funding and/or resources will be sought for supporting new projects or major revisions to existing web education courses.

Action Plan

Once costs and commitments are secured for the planning and implementation of online education, the organization will need to employ and deploy its production capabilities to support its strategy of creating the online course. In order to exist and thrive in a dynamic environment such as distance or online education, the commitment to resources must be addressed by individuals at the strategic (long-term), tactical (intermediate-term), and operational (short-term) levels of the program. Strategic issues are usually broad in nature, addressing questions like the following: How will the program be created? Where are physical and virtual offices for those involved? When should more capacity be added? Thus, by necessity, the time frame for strategic planning and commitment to planning is long-term. Decisions at this level impact the organization's long-range effectiveness in addressing the needs of the online customers. Thus, for the organization to be successful, both commitment and long-range planning must be in alignment with the organization's strategy.

Tactical planning primarily addresses how to efficiently schedule materials and labor within the constraints of the previously made strategic decisions. These tactical decisions, in turn, become the operating constraints under which operational planning and control decisions are made. Lastly, operational planning is narrow and short-term in nature. Issues at this level include the following: What tasks have priority? To whom are the tasks assigned? (Chase, Aquilano, & Jacobs, 1998).

An example is provided to further explain these concepts. As part of the strategic plan at the University of Maryland, specific programs within the Masters' curriculum were planned to be web-based education. To prepare for this implementation, a schedule of implementation was created for the courses, including the person, or champion, responsible for the project and the specific semester for implementation. Specifically, Course 701, a nursing research class, was scheduled to be web-based/online for Fall Semester 2004. Thus, in planning for Course 701, a champion was assigned and given additional time in his or her workload schedule (summer 2004) in order to complete the task of creating the web-based course. The tactical plan began early in the summer semester. The champion, who was a faculty member, arranged for a series of meetings with the course coordinator, the instructional designer engineer, and the multimedia technician in order to plan Course 701. In essence, the faculty members described the material that needed to be communicated to the learners, and the instructional designer was able to provide options as to the best methods for the delivery of that material. Options would include self-learning materials, discussion board, video streaming, or animation. The translation of the traditional classroom to the web is truly a language interpretation process where faculty interacts with instructional design engineers in order to produce a product that meets the needs of the learner and the instructor. This dynamic process is a critical piece to the success of the online course. Lastly, an operational plan was created. This entailed a more technical component of scheduling: which faculty was responsible for which module; which engineer would work with which faculty member; which media specialist would stream the video. Again, each part (strategic, tactic, and operational) is critical to the success of the end product.

DEVELOPMENT PHASE OF ONLINE PROGRAMS

As demonstrated, the commitment to web-based education must be present and on all levels of planning in order for the program to be successful. With that in mind, the development phase of web-based education is now discussed.

Early in the project development phase, priorities need to be determined. Identifying a decision tree for assigning priorities will help to keep the project development team moving forward. This does not have to be complex in nature or created from scratch. It can be as simple as a few sentences, such as, "In line with the school's mission, strategic plan, and the finite number of resources available, priorities will be assigned to new and existing projects." These priorities will assist in workload management and resources allocation decisions. When appropriate and possible, outside funding and/or workload resources will be sought for supporting new projects or major revisions to existing web education courses. An example of priorities for web-based education might be as follows:

1. Maintaining courses that are currently online (web-based, hybrid, or web-enhanced) in a quality manner through evaluation, assessment, and a routine procedure for updating.
2. Bringing up programs and courses (web-based, hybrid, or web-enhanced) that are fully funded from grant or other funding sources.
3. Redesigning courses (traditional courses that are now web-enhanced) that have large learner numbers. The redesign would be to achieve reduction in cost, decrease faculty workload, and address specific learner needs.
4. Bringing up courses or programs (web-based, hybrid, or web-enhanced) with partial funding and a plan that shows potential for income.

Focus of the Development Plan

As with any organization, the core services that customers desire are products and services that are customized to their needs. Thus, the focus of a development plan for web-based education is the customers. Interestingly enough, customers of web-based education involve two groups: the learners and the educators. Keeping this in mind, the starting point for any infrastructure and program development discussion for web-based education should consist of three specific entities:

1. The rationale or basis for the program. (What is the purpose of the program? Who is championing its cause?)
2. The identification of the organization environment. (Where will the program and structure live?)
3. The existing resources necessary and committed to the program. (What capital, personnel, and operational resources are needed for this program to succeed?)

An example of this is the RN to BSN program at the University of Maryland School of Nursing. The RN to BSN program was started in order to meet a market need. Many traditional RNs had voiced their desire to obtain a BSN, but due to work and family constraints, they were unable to attend classes in the traditional manner. After many attempts of Saturday or weekend classes, it was determined that web-based education was the answer. Many of the administrators at the School of Nursing felt that offering the RN to BSN was on the cutting edge of technology and supported this type of program. Currently, over 100 learners are enrolled in the RN to BSN web-based program. Interestingly enough, according to course statistics, most RN to BSN learners are online between the hours of 9 p.m. and 1 a.m. Logistically, this is the time in which work and family commitments have been met, and the learner has time to participate in his or her educational experience. This demonstrates how a program can truly meet the needs of the customer: the learner. Because of the success of this program, the School of Nursing has committed its resources to the program. Changes within the traditional RN to BSN program must also be reflected in the web-based program.

The model presented here offers a method to gather needed information and evaluate the differences in organizations. Some organizations will be required to include faculty salaries, learner tuition, facility expenses, or infrastructure costs in planning and budgeting for programs, while others will not. The traditional business plans often employed by organizations to evaluate its state are difficult to use with the educational endeavor of web-based education. However, by drawing out the common elements all programs have to consider for both the physical and virtual requirements for the learners, faculty, and organization and deliberately addressing them in all four phases (design, development, delivery, and maintenance), an organization can help ensure a successful and quality project.

As presented earlier, the identification of the organization's environment in which the web-based program and structure will exist involves the commitment of the organization. This is demonstrated through the organization's mission, goals and values statements, the strategic plan with web-based education plans, and/or growth information that underpins the program and the organization, the stakeholders, and budget focus. Because the end product is education, the education–learner relationship is core, but the relationship of education to the organization, its parent organization, and the community cannot be overlooked. This supports the idea of collecting and including organizational data. For example, the parent organization's resources may assist in increasing (or decreasing) program costs. A school program starting to offer online courses for continuing education discovers the campus will not grant permission for outsiders to enter the web server or use the e-mail system unless they are registered with the school. This involves a separate fee that the learners must pay. How are the registration and method of payment to be handled? Can the current registrar provide the services to accommodate the additional learners? The extent to which current resources are being used and how much additional workload they can tolerate must be determined prior to assuming they can indeed support the new workload requirements or costs. Additional questions include the following:

- Is there server space to hold new course management software? Are upgrades necessary, and what are the costs of the upgrades?
- Are there enough staff currently working the help desk to support the additional learner and faculty questions?
- Is the instructional technologist and/or web specialist and/or computer specialist workload able to be increased, or will additional personnel be needed and where would they come from?

● How will resources be shared across departments and among supervisors? Who will hire, supervise, or manage the additional instructional technologist or server or server manager? Where will they or it be located?

Evaluation Plan

As with any program, evaluation of the web-based program is critical. Evaluation involves assessing the strengths and weaknesses of a program to ensure that the program is meeting the goals and objectives that it set out to meet. The development plan must include the critical information that maximizes the success of web-based education, as well as the success of the organization. Graves (2004) posited the following guidelines an organization may use in order to evaluate the success of a program or offering:

● The scope and scale of the offering and identification of the learning technology players.
● Budget planning to include full project, lifetime budget oversight and refinement including information and learning technology representation.
● Funding that is truly life cycle inclusive and not a one-time amount.
● Computer access that is both reliable and affordable to the user.
● Attention to controlling costs through the conscious centralization of services or cost sharing.
● Building the necessary infrastructure with the focus on the learner and instructor (internal and external customers).
● Using a variety of roles in the development, implementation, and maintenance of web-based education, such as content expert, instructional design, computer support, program manager, and so on.

As an organization is able to match these guidelines, the more successful the program or offering will be. Additionally, the organization needs to consider the integration, or sharing, of resources across the organization and its environment, as illustrated in Figure 2.2. What this means is that a number of systems can work together, share information, and act as one system toward the user. For example, the University of Maryland School of Nursing would consider the integration of resources across the school itself, within the university system, and within the community at large. Again, when an organization is able to maximize its resources, the more successful the program or offering will be.

Through this analysis, information from both the physical and virtual world aspects for online programs or courses will be identified. This information will assist in the planning, building, and operations of the infrastructure in support of this type of educational endeavor. Often, these virtual foundations, policies and procedures, and/or additional costs are often overlooked or considered only after the fact or as problems arise. Once the integration of resources has occurred, the organization may determine that potential overlapping of supports and resources may develop (Figure 2.3). For example, a computer help desk at the school level may be a duplication in services if a computer help desk exists on the university level. Thus, once these duplications have

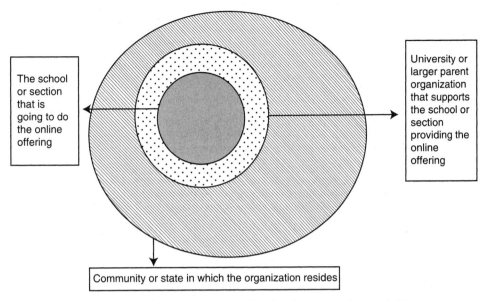

The school or section that is going to do the online offering

University or larger parent organization that supports the school or section providing the online offering

Community or state in which the organization resides

FIGURE 2.2 Integration of resources across school, university, and community.

been identified, the pooling of resources among the school, university, and community should be addressed in order to minimize cost and maximize efficiency for all involved.

The ultimate goal for a web-based program is equal worlds for the learners and the faculty. This means the same services and amenities are present in both physical and virtual worlds (Figure 2.4). If learner registration, advising, financial aid services, counseling, faculty office hours, library services, and bookstore services are present in the physical world, there should be some form of the same services in the virtual world. As the number of courses or programs move toward online offerings, the more significant

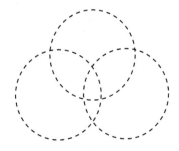

Potentially overlapping supports and resources (e.g., computer help desk may be at parent organization level for the school or section doing the actual online teaching)

FIGURE 2.3 Potential overlapping of identified resources.

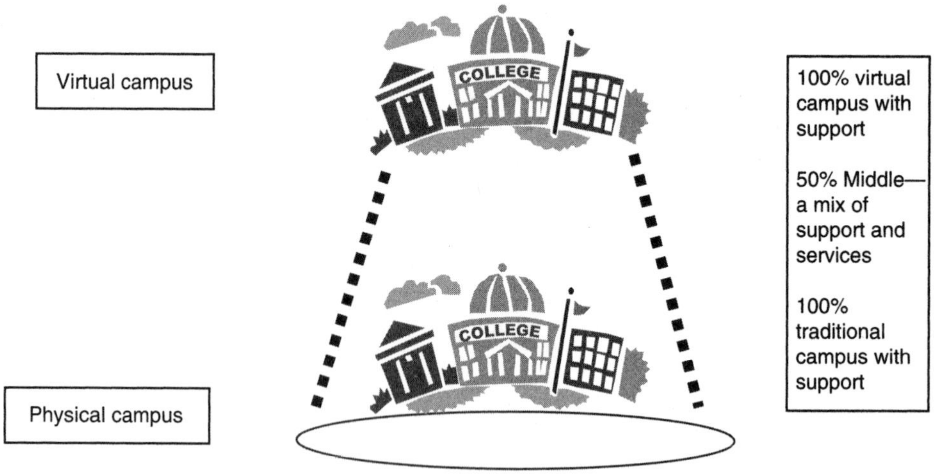

FIGURE 2.4 Equal worlds: virtual and physical campuses.

technology infrastructure and online services need to become. Once services exist in both settings, the same questions on capacity may need to be addressed.

In the measurement of success of the web-based program, web-based courses face the same types of review as the traditional classroom courses. Learners, instructors, administrators, and information technologists should participate in the ongoing process of evaluation. Progress of the web-based courses will be made through the information and insight that evaluation brings. As part of every web-based course, learners and instructors should be asked to complete a survey. The survey should focus on questions that reflect the style and nature of the course. For example, a sample survey may include the following types (to be answered with a Likert scale of Strongly Disagree, Disagree, Neutral, Agree, or Strongly Agree):

● Was the use of multimedia (audio, video, graphics, or animations) effective in conveying the course content?
● Were the online support resources helpful?
● Were the required electronic library resources adequate and readily available online?
● Did the use of technology enhance my overall learning experience?

From these types of questions, progress will be made in changing and adapting the web-based program to reflect the needs of the learners and the educators. It is important to keep in mind that progress is often made in gradual stages, by incremental improvements.

Capacity

In order to assess for the needs of the customers, an organization must be aware of the necessary elements needed for a web-based program to be successful. It is important to keep in mind that the goal of the web-based program is to provide learners with greater access to education and to better accommodate the large population of nontraditional students (Hartman & Truman-Davis, 2001). In order to accommodate this, organizations must identify those elements. A sample listing of the infrastructure elements necessary for a web-based program are listed below. It is important to keep in mind that as the scope, scale, and support of the program changes, many of the infrastructure elements may also change and may be eliminated. For example, if learners are physically coming to campus, processes such as registration, recruiting and/or marketing, library resources, admissions, bookstore, and advising could be offered in the traditional manner as compared to virtual offering. However, if learners were not physically coming to campus, these entities would need to be addressed in terms of online access and online processes for the project. Additionally, other access and service methods would need to be identified in order to provide the online learners similar educational experiences as the traditional learners receive. The necessary elements to examine include the following:

● *Personnel:* Faculty (content experts for both developing and teaching online), instructional designer for all phases of development to maintenance and evaluation, web specialist/administrator, network/computer specialist (may also be IT help desk), program coordinator, learner services supports (registration, admissions, advising, counseling, library, bookstore, and so on). It is important to recognize that as online education moves from the traditional, to the web-enhanced, to web-centric to web-based, the need for additional personnel and supportive staff increases (Figure 2.5). Organizations should be aware of the increased needs as online programs grow and develop.

● *Activities:* Program and course development, course administration, faculty and team member training (course development, transition to online teaching, delivering and managing courses online, copyright and intellectual property in the digital age including the TEACH Act, building learner communities and services online, evaluation of program and courses at a minimum).

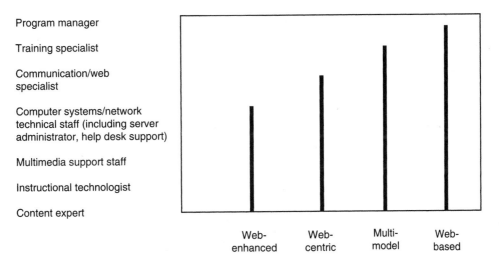

FIGURE 2.5 Members of the team by type of online education.

● *Services:* Marketing and recruiting, registration, admissions, advising, counseling, library, bookstore, semester orientation of faculty and learners to resources such as hardware, software, courseware, and library services.

● *Hardware and software:* Course management software (homegrown or commercial, like Blackboard, WebCT), web server, course management server, database server, multimedia server, electronic backup and/or storage devices, streaming video server, e-mail software and server if not included in the courseware package; electronic grade book if not in course management package, communication channels, stand-alone assets and software (course development applications like Dreamweaver) or networked computers and printers for the development team content expert; web specialist, instructional designer, computer/network specialist, program manager, learner services, and so on. Similar to that of personnel, the dependency on hardware and software increases as online education moves from the traditional, to the web-enhanced, to web-centric to web-based (Figure 2.6).

● *Indirect costs:* Administrative overhead (office space for faculty and support personnel for learners and faculty, consumable supplies including duplication, ink, paper, pens, and others); copyright and electronic library costs including electronic reserve support; digitalization of videos for webcasts; faculty training that includes teaching them to plan for times when the technology fails, and release time for development and evaluation; faculty stipend for teaching online; image and photograph costs for permissions; security software and/or monitoring; data communication charges for lines into the organization and throughout the organization connecting the team personnel; server space; backup costs including tapes, disaster recovery planning and off-site storage of tapes; archival costs for courses; copyright, licensing, or patenting of product; travel of faculty and paying for proctors off-site for proctored testing; evaluation software; peer or user group expenses in time, room, and administrative

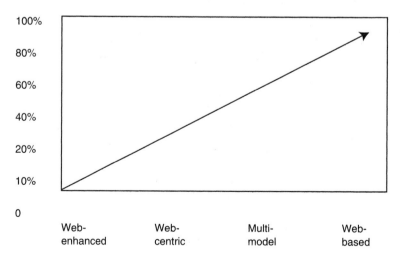

FIGURE 2.6 Dependency on functioning hardware and software by type of online education.

support; advertising; turnover rates of faculty; retention rate for learners; and, how many faculty and learners are experienced online participants.

● *Revenue:* Revenue represents the amount earned by an organization; that is, the actual or expected cash inflows received due to the organization's major business of providing a product or service. In terms of web-based education, revenue is generated from tuition and learners' fees in exchange for access to the educational experience. Depending on the type of organization, revenues may be generated from a number of sources, including the learner tuition for a web-based class, technological-based fees for access to specialized programs or seminars, or flat rate fees for special one-time, continuing educational programs. Thus, in the phases of planning and developing, the organization can project potential revenue sources based on the program offering that is available through the organization. For example, if enrollment or attendance figures are known, then revenue can be easily projected. Another source of revenue for the organization lies in developmental or start-up funds. This type of revenue is geared toward the initial cost of development and implementation. Every organization is different and has its own specific revenue needs; however, it is important for an organization to identify all the costs that will be accrued at start-up. Revenues for developing the course offering (start-up funds) and then supporting the course offerings (ongoing revenue) must be closely considered and monitored (Baker and Baker, 2004; Penner, 2004). An excellent resource outlining the specific costs for start-up and sustainability for online learning is "Is Distance Learning Worth It? Helping to Determine the Costs of Online Courses" by Brian M. Morgan of Marshall University. The interactive web site allows individuals to enter in costs and create a full spreadsheet projection of costs. A sample spreadsheet is provided in Figure 2.7.

Needs Assessment

In order for the organization to organize and process the information that is necessary to develop and maintain a successful online program, a needs assessment is provided as a resource tool in Box 2.1 in order to assist in identifying what specific information is needed. These needs must be examined in relation to the organization's goals and demands for the online efforts. Again, this must be reflected in the mission and vision statements of the organization. The more in agreement the two lists are (goals and demands plus resources), the better the chance for program success both initially and over time. Care must be taken to be realistic and identify if the resources are present, as well as whether they are currently committed to other programs. To ensure effective implementation, evaluation procedures for the project and course offering need to be built in at the planning stage (Williams, Paprock, & Covington, 1999).

In today's environment, organizations are learning to operate more efficiently, working more with less; adding additional workload to current workload may overextend existing operations. The more information known about current workload and the potential workload (demands of the new program), the more accurate and realistic the assessments and estimates can be in order to achieve implementation and sustainability (Novotny & Corbett, 2000).

Category	Year 1	Year 2	Year 3	Year 4	Year 5	Year 6	Year 7	Cumulative
DEVELOPMENTAL COSTS based on a Growth Rate of 20%								
Courses Being Developed	12	2	3	3	4	5	6	35
Stipend for Development	$0.00	$0.00	$0.00	$0.00	$0.00	$0.00	$0.00	$0.00
Hidden Costs								
Supplies Consumed	$1,800.00	$300.00	$450.00	$450.00	$600.00	$750.00	$900.00	$5,250.00
Faculty Development								
Faculty Training	$2,188.80	$364.80	$547.20	$547.20	$729.60	$912.00	$1,094.40	$6,384.00
Instructional Technology Support	$9,192.96	$1,532.16	$2,298.24	$2,298.24	$3,064.32	$3,830.40	$4,596.48	$26,812.80
Library Support	$1,193.09	$198.85	$298.27	$298.27	$397.70	$497.12	$596.54	$3,479.84
TEACHING COSTS								
Learner Enrollments	0	600	700	850	1000	1200	1450	5800
Stipends for Teaching	$0.00	$0.00	$0.00	$0.00	$0.00	$0.00	$0.00	$0.00
Hidden Costs								
Office Space	$2,611.20	$5,657.60	$6,745.60	$8,051.20	$9,574.40	$11,532.80	$13,926.40	$58,099.20
Administrative Overheads	$0.00	$11,544.00	$13,468.00	$16,354.00	$19,240.00	$23,088.00	$27,898.00	$111,592.00
Help Desk Support	$0.00	$2,790.72	$3,255.84	$3,953.52	$4,651.20	$5,581.44	$6,744.24	$26,976.96

FIGURE 2.7 Projecting costs of online education. Adapted from http://webpages.marshall.edu/~morgan16/onlinecosts/. Accessed on September 9, 2005.

This planning process continues by analyzing the information gathered to identify the fit or gaps between what currently is present, and what is needed to support the project for three blocks of time: near term (0 to 2 years) development, medium term (2 to 5 years) maintenance, and long term (5 plus years) growth. The resulting plan will have a comprehensive portion that identifies the needed infrastructure for carrying out successful online projects. The plan, once approved by the project team members and adopted by the organization, will need a project manager to oversee the implementation. This person will need a project implementation team with members from the assessment team who represent the major stakeholders and customers. A sample team might include a project sponsor (administration representative with sign off power), procurement officer to interact with vendors and contracts, project or development process manager, content expert or representative instructional (faculty) member who can coordinate with the one or more content experts, and course management software expert or trainer with this knowledge.

Needs Assessment

BOX 2.1

Organization Goals and Demands

1. What are the goals for offering the course or program online?
2. Who are the stakeholders in the course or program?
3. What are the organization's stated beliefs, strategic plans, and goals about distance education?
4. What are the economic and political items influencing the distance education efforts?

Resources

5. What is the number of courses or programs that are now online partially or completely?
6. What is the number of courses or programs that will be online partially or will be completely online?
7. If other programs or courses are online, what was the time required to bring them up? What is the suggested time line for bringing up the course or program?
8. Does the school or parent organization currently support other online courses or programs? If so, what and how does it support the program, learners, and faculty?
9. Does the school or parent organization have clerical and technical support staff that could assist in the program or course development, implementation, maintenance, and learner or faculty training and orientation?
10. What are the computer hardware, operating system, specialty software, and network systems available for the program at the school or parent organization level? Are they currently running any other like programs?
11. What are the computer and network supports available at the school or parent organization? What are the hours of support and are any supports virtually available around the clock , 7 days a week?
12. How many faculty have taught online before or are interested in or available to teach in the program? How many faculty have had orientation and training in online teaching and/or the course management software that is or will be used in the program? Is there currently training available?
13. How many learners who are going to be in the program have been in online courses before?
14. Is computer ownership now a requirement for learners?
15. Is there presently a requirement for learners and faculty to use e-mail for communication?
16. Are any of these systems (learner registration, advising, financial aid advising, counseling, office hours, library services, and bookstore) services now completely electronic and do they talk bidirectional between the school and the parent organization?
17. Does the school or parent organization have distance sites at present and policies and procedures governing learner testing, attendance, online behavior, computer literacy, readiness for taking an online course, and information or communication system literacy?

(continued)

Needs Assessment (continued)

18. Does the school or parent organization currently have distance sites and policies and procedures governing faculty workload for these classes or programs for the development phase, the implementation phase, and for teaching established ones?

19. Does the school or parent organization currently have distance sites and policies and procedures governing patent, copyright and intellectual property ownership for courses and course content? Are there organization resources available to help answer questions related to these issues for the online environment?

CONCLUSION

This chapter presents an overview of the needs assessment, administrative and support requirements, and other essential components necessary to develop and sustain web-based education in an academic environment. As academic institutions look to web-based education as a means of responding to market demand for online education, these entities will be critical in the development and sustainability of a web-based program. As presented, these guidelines are general in nature so that they can be molded to fit the specifics of an individual program. The next chapter will further develop these ideas with a focus on the technological considerations.

■ LEARNING ACTIVITIES

● Apply the information you have learned in this chapter to your current school or work setting by completing the needs assessment tool to the best of your ability at this time.
● Identify your resources needed to complete your needs assessment. Share your results in small groups.

REFERENCES

Baker, J. J., & Baker, R. W. (2004). *Health care finance: Basic tools for nonfinancial managers.* Boston: Jones and Barlett.

Bates, A. W. (2000). *Managing technological change.* San Francisco: Jossey-Bass Publishers.

Bartolic-Zlomislic, S., & Bates, A. W. (1999). Investing in online learning: Potential benefits and limitations. *Canadian Journal of Communication, 24*(3), 349–366.

Billings, D. (2000). A framework for assessing outcomes and practices in Web-based courses in nursing. *Journal of Nursing Education 39*(2):60–67.

Bourne, J., & Moore, J. (Eds.). (2001). *Online education: Learning effectiveness, faculty satisfaction and cost effectiveness.* (Vol. 2). Sloan Center for Online Learning: Needham, MA.

Chase, R. B., Aquilano, N. J., & Jacobs, F. R. (1998). *Production and operations management: Manufacturing and services.* (8th ed.) Boston: Irwin McGraw-Hill.

Cleverly, W. O., & Cameron, A. E. (2003). *Essentials of health care finance.* (5th ed.) Boston: Jones and Barlett.

Daft, R. L. (1998). *Organizational theory and design.* (8th ed) Cincinnati, Ohio: South-Western College Publishing.

Draves, W. A. (2002). *Teaching online.* River Falls, WI: LERN Books.

Graves, W. H. (2004, February). Academic redesign: Accomplishing more with less. *JALN, 8*(1), 26–38. Retrieved August 29, 2005, from http://www.aln.org/publications/jaln/v8n1/pdf/v8n1_graves.pdf

Hartman, J. L., & Truman-Davis, B. (2000). *Factors relating to the satisfaction of faculty teaching on-line course at the University of Central Florida.* In: J. Bourne & J. Moore (Eds.), *Online education: Learning effectiveness, faculty satisfaction and cost effectiveness.* (Vol. 2). Sloan Center for Online Learning: Needham, MA.

Marquis, B. L., & Huston, C. J. (1994). *Management decision making for nurses.* (2nd ed.) Philadelphia: Lippincott Williams & Wilkins.

Meredith, J. R., & Mantel, S. J. (2000). *Project management: A managerial approach.* (5th ed.) New York: John Wiley & Sons.

Morgan, B. M. (2005). Is distance learning worth it? Helping to determine the cost of online courses. Retrieved August 29, 2005, from http://webpages.marshall.edu/~morgan16/onlinecosts/

Novotny, J., & Corbett, C. (2000). Nurse practitioner education: The Virginia experience. In J. Novotny (Ed.). *Distance education in nursing.* (pp 153–179) New York: Springer Publishing.

O'Neil, C. A., Fisher, C. A., & Newbold, S. K. (2004). *Developing an online course: Best practices for nurse educators.* New York: Springer Publishing Company, Inc.

Penner, S. J. (2004) *Introduction to health care economics and financial management.* Philadelphia: Lippincott Williams & Wilkins.

Phillips, J. J. (1994). *Measuring return on investment: Volume I.* Alexandria, VA: American Society for Training and Development.

Phillips, P. P. (2002). *The bottomline of ROI: Basics, benefits, and barriers to measuring training and performance improvement.* Atlanta, GA: CEP Press.

Simonson, M., Smaldino, S., Albright, M., & Zvacek, S. (2003). *Teaching and learning at a distance: foundations of distance education.* Upper Saddle River, NJ: Merrill Prentice Hall.

Ward, W. J. (1994). *Health care budgeting and financial management for non-financial managers.* Westport, CT: Auburn House.

Whalen, T., & Wright, D. (1999). *Business process reengineering for the use of distance learning at Bell Canada.* Hershey, PA: Idea Group.

Williams, M., Paprock, K., & Covington, B. (1999). *Distance learning: The essential guide.* Thousand Oaks, CA: Sage Publications.

Objectives

Upon completion of this chapter, the learner will be able to:

- Describe the roles and responsibilities of information and instructional technologists for implementing online education offerings.
- Analyze the necessary system requirements for hosting and providing online education services.
- Evaluate the key features of courseware management systems and development tools that will best meet their needs.
- Develop appropriate end-user requirements for successful user engagement, as well as virtual mechanisms for training and technical support.

Key Terms

Courseware: Software applications that facilitate the management and distribution of instructional materials, enable students to interact with and discuss learning materials, and provide ways to assess mastery of desired learning outcomes.

Information Technology: The study, application, and processing of data, and the development and use of the hardware, software, and procedures associated with this processing.

Instructional Technology: The systemic and systematic application of strategies and techniques derived from behavioral, cognitive, and constructivist theories to the solution of instructional problems.

Open Source: Software applications that users have the freedom to copy, use, and modify, provided that any newly developed source code is shared with others, the original license and copyright is not modified or removed, and derivative works apply the same license.

Peripherals: External devices that can be connected to a computer, such as a printer or scanner.

Storyboards: A panel or series of panels on which a set of sketches using pictures, numbers, and words is arranged depicting clearly and consecutively the important changes of scene and action in a series of shots in order of occurrence, which taken together tell an interesting story.

CHAPTER THREE

Technological Considerations

NOLA STAIR, SAVITHRAMMA SANJOY, AND SHELLEY JORDON

Chapter Outline

D elivering high quality online instruction requires a robust and well-coordinated environment that will meet the varying technological needs of administrators, faculty, staff, and students. In Chapter One of this text, a general framework for online education was presented (Figure 1.2). In this chapter, the technological considerations, which guide the development of the technological infrastructure and the course-specific requirements presented in Figure 1.2, are addressed.

Traditional campus networks are often expected by administration, faculty, and students to fully support the delivery requirements of web-based distance education; this expectation may be unrealistic in a time of rapid change in technological capabilities.

Certain campus environments may be inadequate and unable to support a growing number of remote users. Depending on the number of online courses or programs, mix of instructional content and multimedia strategies, and asynchronous or synchronous communication modes that are to be offered, it may be more economical to arrange partnerships with Application Service Providers (ASP) to guarantee an appropriate level of service (McAlister, Rivera, & Hallam, 2005).

Regardless of whether the delivery system for web-based distance education will be provided through one's campus network or outsourced, this chapter will focus on the critical success factors, rather than detailed technical issues, that pertain to the development of a collaborative and reliable technology infrastructure.

WORKING WITH INFORMATION AND INSTRUCTIONAL TECHNOLOGISTS

The roles of today's technology professionals are increasingly diverse, and it is important to understand the unique contributions that each technology group can offer in the development and ongoing sustainability of any distance education project. Although the actual hardware and network configuration ultimately provides the connectivity between people and places, the personnel who operate behind the scenes are often overlooked.

Information Technology Staff

Typically, the campus information technology staff manages the day-to-day responsibilities of supporting desktop computers, maintaining enterprise servers, and managing the campus network. In addition, this group is responsible for diagnosing and analyzing hardware, software, and telecommunications problems that are submitted to the campus help desk. As a result, information technologists will be able to assist with the following tasks:

- Identifying resources and constraints of the delivery environment.
- Analyzing hardware requirements for supporting courseware applications.
- Establishing adequate, incremental, and periodic full backup procedures.
- Troubleshooting technical difficulties and provide solutions.

Instructional Technology Staff

Although instructional technology staff may assist with implementing technical systems and troubleshooting problems, they are primarily responsible for "the systemic and systematic application of strategies and techniques derived from behavioral, cognitive, and constructivist theories to the solution of instructional problems" (AECT, 2005, p. 1). Therefore, instructional technologists will be able to assist with the following tasks:

- Identifying resources and constraints of the development environment.
- Conducting a content analysis of instructional materials for courses.
- Developing flowcharts, storyboards, and templates to identify key learning concepts that need to be reconceptualized for online delivery.
- Designing and enhancing course materials to accommodate various learning styles with a variety of instructional and multimedia strategies.

Both information and instructional technologists should be involved with the development of the campus distance learning strategic plan. A collaborative decision-making and planning process will help identify potential strengths, weaknesses, opportunities, and threats that will ultimately impact the offering of a web-based distance education program.

The distance learning strategic plan should include and clearly address identified roles of responsibility and communication channels, network and server reliability and user connectivity issues, hardware storage devices and backup procedures, use of courseware development applications, procedures for maintenance notification, infrastructure capacity for growth, and provision of technical support for both faculty and students.

General Hardware Requirements

A distributed network infrastructure is the core of delivering online instruction and consists of three functional layers: physical, network, and applications. The first two layers involve the transportation of electronic signals and devices, while the third layer deals with application services (Long, 2000). The Internet connects users to a variety of applications and resources for online instruction.

To provide a working system for web-based distance learning, there are many hardware and software requirements for both the application servers and the client (faculty and/or student) machines. As shown in Figure 3.1, there is a need for individual servers to host the course management system, course management database, collection of multimedia objects, and e-mail system for asynchronous communication. This constitutes the minimum hardware for setting up a functional distance-learning environment.

Each server consists of both hardware and software components. The selection of server operating systems includes Windows, UNIX, Solaris, or Linux. Many of the course management systems are designed and developed for Windows-based servers; however, some course management systems are specifically designed and built to run on

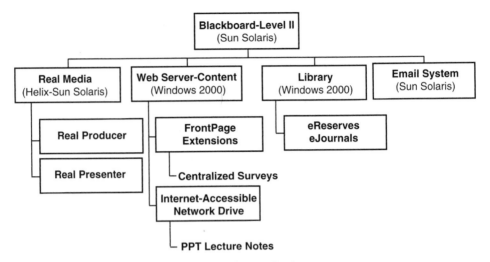

FIGURE 3.1 Network diagram and supporting applications.

the other server operating systems mentioned above. Minimum suggested server configurations include the following:

- Hard disk space—at least 20 gigabytes (GB) for ongoing storage.
- Memory—at least 2GB of random access memory (RAM).
- Processor speed—at least Pentium III 900 Megahertz (Mhz).

The hardware configuration of the course management system server will depend on the number of users and types of asynchronous or synchronous applications (chat rooms, discussion boards, file exchanges, online exams, quizzes, surveys, and so on) that will be hosted by the server. Most course management applications will specify the minimum hardware requirements based on the number of users (in thousands) and also based on two, or even three, servers.

A combination of servers is necessary in order to dedicate each server to host one application, such as the course management application itself, a database server as a back end to the course management application for storage and retrieval purposes, and a media server to host multimedia objects. For example:

Database servers serve as a supplement and back end to the course management application. They hold and/or store all the instructional and academic records content of an online course. Depending on the course content, the online course may contain a variety of different file formats such as text files, spreadsheets, presentation files, graphics, audio, and video files. These multimedia files might be stored in the database server or on a separate multimedia server.

Multimedia servers are used to hold and/or store streaming multimedia content, such as audio and video files. It is recommended to have a separate multimedia server because the multimedia files tend to be of larger size. Instructional technologists might have to store multimedia files in a variety of different formats, which requires double or triple the storage space. Files are stored in different formats, so that end users are not restricted to using a single application program to view the files. Also, the end user might not have access to have a high speed network or Internet connectivity.

E-mail servers provide the most convenient, important, and widely used media to communicate between all the parties involved in an online course. Although there are other ways to communicate, e-mail is the preferred way of students to communicate specific questions to the instructor. E-mail capabilities may be integrated within the course management system, connected to the university's external e-mail program from the course management tool, or connected to the user's personal e-mail system.

The software component consists of the server's operating system, the course management application, and any other applications or programs that support or provide enhancements to the online learning experience. These applications may be needed to extend the course management application's functionality and might be built-in or external to the course management application. For example, such additional applications might include full-featured discussion board or e-mail systems (both asynchronous communications tools) and chat rooms or messaging devices (synchronous communicating tools through which text, voice, or video messages are exchanged between all the parties instantaneously).

Collaborative Planning and Decision Making

Even with the most reliable network infrastructure, technology recovery plans should be established with specific policies and procedures that include the following:

- Retention of academic records from courseware management system.
- Notification and prevention of unauthorized dissemination of electronic work.
- Submission deadlines for assignments or exams delayed due to power outages.

An institutional collaboration with information and instructional technologists is a critical success factor for establishing a distributed network infrastructure that will support the implementation and ongoing maintenance of a web-based distance learning program. As enrollment grows, ongoing planning and decision making must continue to be addressed in order to ensure adequate hardware and software, infrastructure stability, and instructional and technical support for scalability purposes.

SELECTING COURSEWARE MANAGEMENT APPLICATIONS

Courseware management systems facilitate the management and distribution of instructional materials, enable students to interact with and discuss learning materials, and provide ways to assess mastery of desired learning outcomes. Figure 3.2 provides an example of how instructional materials can be displayed in a courseware management system. Students are able to access the materials by selecting the appropriate options from the courseware management system's navigation bar, as depicted on the left-hand side of Figure 3.2. During the selection process of an institution's courseware management system, it is important to recognize that some systems are

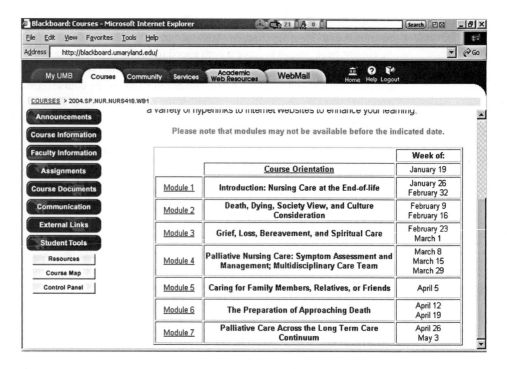

FIGURE 3.2 Screenshot of End of Life course in courseware management system. © 2004 University of Maryland School of Nursing.

distinguished in terms of administrative productivity and ease of use, while others are noted for their complex academic-related features. However, many lack sophisticated data analysis and reporting tools for drill-down reporting and statistical analysis (Olsen, 2001).

Factors for Consideration

The cost of courseware systems can range from no cost to expensive solutions. There are two methods in which an organization can implement a course management system. Depending on the campus capability and competence for handling the design, development, maintenance, and administration of the required hardware and software, campuses may choose to handle everything in-house or outsource the entire service to an outside ASP. An ASP model would manage all software installations, redundant and conditioned power supplies, round-the-clock help desk assistance and monitoring, nightly tape back-ups, and a secure facility.

Regardless, the selection of a courseware management system (either commercial or open source) should consider a range of institutional viewpoints, such as infrastructure requirements, faculty and/or student input regarding the availability and use of features, and integration capabilities with existing student and financial information systems.

Key Features and Tools

From a functional perspective, a courseware management system is defined partly by features they should and should not include (Leslie, 2003). The working definition of course management systems excludes single function software (i.e., stand-alone assessment tools, such as QuestionMark; synchronous tools, such as WebBoard; or authoring packages, such as Authorware) that does not have features or tools for:

- Providing opportunities for both synchronous and asynchronous student participation with the instructional content, with other students, and with the instructor.
- Facilitating multiple aspects of course design and content management.
- Administering assessments and tracking usage from various perspectives.
- Structuring content delivery and course progression.

As depicted in Figure 3.2, courseware management systems should provide the following key capabilities:

- Posting of announcements and updates for student viewing.
- Provision of full (or limited) access to:
  - Course information, such as the syllabus and assignments.
  - Contact information about course instructor, technical support, and development team.
  - Detailed module content and supporting materials, web sites, etc.
- Delivery of exams, quizzes, or surveys.
- Communication via synchronous and asynchronous methods—e-mail, chat rooms, and discussion boards.
- Enabling students with tools to submit assignments and/or check grades.

Cost–Benefit Analysis

A final cost–benefit analysis will help determine which courseware management system meets the institutional needs for online instruction. The Western Cooperative for Educational Telecommunications (WCET) developed EduTools, which can assist colleges and universities with analyzing and comparing various courseware management systems. Available course management systems and their web sites are listed in Table 3.1.

Tools such as EduTools can assist with distinguishing between the various types of systems available for the various educational needs of offering web-based distance education. It is important to know the difference between course management systems and other commercially available systems (Leslie, 2003):

Courseware management system (CMS)—focused on the display and maintenance of content (announcements, assignments, assessments, and communications) with limited or no pedagogical tools for creating content.

Learning management system (LMS)—typically aimed at corporate training and functionally more focused on learner tracking and competency management.

Learning content management system (LCMS)—most often found in corporate settings and typically used to create and/or manage learning content or learning objects that are accessible to learners anytime, anywhere.

Course Management Systems

TABLE 3.1	COMPANY	WEB SITE
	Angel	http://www.cyberlearninglabs.com
	Blackboard	http://www.blackboard.com
	Desire2Learn	http://www.desire2learn.com/
	Ecollege	http://www.ecollege.com
	Educator	http://www.ucompass.com
	Jenzabar	http://www.jenzabar.com
	LearnWise	http://www.learnwise.com/
	WebCT	http://www.webct.com

Products aimed at the K–12 market—share some aspect with CMSs but address additional audiences and interoperate with different back-end systems.

Open Source Options

Some courseware management systems are distributed freely as open source under the GNU General Public License. The GNU General Public License is designed to provide users with the freedom to copy, use, and modify the courseware management system, provided that additional source code is shared with others, the original license and copyright is not modified or removed, and derivative works apply the same license.

It is important to emphasize that many commercial courseware management systems were not designed for pedagogical development of instructional materials. Open source projects, such as Whiteboard (http://whiteboard.sourceforge.net) or Moodle (http://moodle.org), are part of ongoing research and development efforts designed to support pedagogical delivery. A compilation of open-source courseware management systems with specific details, such as developer, country of origin, license type, and notes, is available online at EduTools' web site.

DEVELOPING CONTENT AND APPROPRIATE SOFTWARE TOOLS

Once a courseware management system has been selected, the next major step is the authoring and development of content. When reconceptualizing courses for online delivery, it is critical to have a well thought-out instructional design plan. The e-learning movement and the supporting instructional theories are still in the early stages of maturity. However, one important lesson learned is that existing models for traditional classroom instruction do not always translate directly online.

Instructional Design Concepts

Sound instructional design should incorporate the following ideas:

- ● *Display of content*—What is the most effective medium to display, introduce, and support instructional content? People learn differently.
- ● *Keep it simple*—Determine the most important issues:
  - ● Managing content size and sequence.
  - ● Selecting appropriate examples to illustrate key concepts.
  - ● Allowing users time to integrate and process concepts before proceeding to the next level.
- ● *Use of medium*—What multiple modalities can be used to facilitate learning?

Use of Multimedia and Engaging the Learner

The exponential growth of web-based distance education creates a breeding ground for new teaching strategies. One such strategy is infusing multimedia into the learning environment. Multimedia is a sequential or simultaneous use of a variety of media formats in a single presentation or program (Newby, Stepich, Lehman, & Russell, 2000). It involves any combination of text and graphics and/or images, streaming audio or video, animation or simulations, and software programs. In order to navigate the power of this medium in education successfully, faculty must be trained not only to use technology but also to shift the ways in which they organize and deliver material. First, teachers must buy into the philosophy that multimedia technology can enhance student learning. In addition, this shift can increase the potential for learners to take charge of their own learning process and facilitate the development of a sense of community among the learners (Palloff & Pratt, 2001).

According to dual coding theory (Najjar, 1996), information is processed through one of two generally independent channels. One channel processes verbal information, such as text or audio. The other channel processes nonverbal images such as illustrations and sounds in the environment. Information can be processed through both channels. Information processing through both channels is called referential processing and has an additive effect on recall (Najjar, 1996). Learning is better when the information is referentially processed through two channels than when the information is processed through only one channel. Referential processing may produce this additive effect because the learner creates more cognitive paths that can be followed to retrieve the information. Table 3.2 offers suggestions as to how media can be used to augment instructional objectives.

According to Robert Gagne or Madeline Hunter's events of instruction (Gagne & Briggs, 1979; Hunter, 1982) in Table 3.3, one must first grab the attention of the learner. Hunter believes in opening class with a short activity or prompt that focuses on the students' attention before the actual lesson. Multimedia technology provides effective attention-gathering tools, which can be used to enrich and complement classroom teaching and learning and may even reinvent subject matter (Brace & Roberts, 1996; Wise & Groom, 1996).

A new educational technology delivery tool deserves considerations of new teaching methods. Simply transferring text onto a computer screen is not using the potential of online instruction to its full capacity, especially for today's diverse learning styles and

Empirically Supported Suggestions for Allocating Media

TABLE 3.2	INFORMATION TO BE LEARNED	SUGGESTED MEDIA
	Assembly instructions	Text with supported pictures
	Procedural information	Explanatory text with diagrams or animation
	Problem solving	Animation with explanatory verbal narration
	Recognition	Graphics or images
	Spatial	Graphics or images
	Small amounts of verbal for a short time	Streaming audio or video; narrated animation; simulation
	Story details	Streaming audio or video with soundtrack (text with supportive illustration)

student characteristics. That is why the use of multimedia is so valuable in the learning process. For example, as depicted in Figure 3.3, the listing of procedural information often consists of explanatory text. However, the learner's understanding of these procedures can be enhanced with specific diagrams or animations that help clarify key concepts.

Digital Libraries and Digital Collections

Institutions should consider the availability (or unavailability) of library resources for students taking online courses. Ideally, catalogs, databases, journals, and full-text newspapers should be password-protected and accessible electronically via the Internet. However, electronic access to databases or journals may or may not be included in the cost of regular print subscriptions. In addition, the ability to access articles may be limited, or

Events of Instruction

TABLE 3.3	GAGNE AND BRIGGS	HUNTER
	Gaining attention	Review
	Informing learner of objective	Anticipatory set
	Stimulating recall	Objectives and purpose
	Describing material	Input and modeling
	Eliciting desired behavior	Checking for understanding
	Providing feedback	Guided practice
	Assessing the behavior	Independent practice

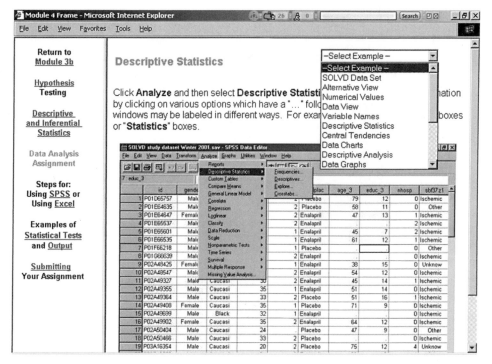

FIGURE 3.3 Screenshot of procedural instructions in nursing research course. © 2004 University of Maryland School of Nursing.

additional fees may be charged for students to download them. Therefore, library information specialists should be included in the distance-learning strategic planning process.

　　If funding is an issue, joining a library consortium is one way to expand one's electronic offerings. Also, there are a growing number of freely available electronic journals, such as the following:

● *Directory of Open Access Journals:* http://www.doaj.org
● *Free Medical Journals:* http://www.freemedicaljournals.com
● *HighWire Press,* Internet Imprint of the Stanford University Libraries: http://highwire.stanford.edu1

　　Finally, on many campuses, the traditional course reserve list has been replaced by the use of password-protected electronic reserves, or commonly known as e-reserves (Figure 3.4), where students can view, print, or download resources in which copyright clearance has been requested and granted.

PROVIDING STUDENT REQUIREMENTS, TRAINING, AND TECHNICAL SUPPORT

Academic health science centers often have high speed networks that transmit data much faster than a dial-up modem. When authoring and developing content for online delivery,

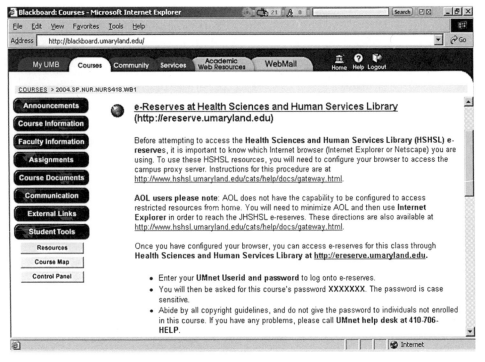

FIGURE 3.4 Screenshot of e-Reserves process for students. © 2004 University of Maryland School of Nursing.

it is critical to keep the end user's minimum technology requirements in mind. Therefore, one should:

● Set minimum standards for accessing online materials.
● Develop materials that are consistent with minimum standards.
● Constantly test developed materials from the minimum standards.
● Inform students well in advance when exceeding minimum standards.

Personal Computer Hardware and Software

Students should have a workstation equipped with the hardware and software recommended by the institution offering online education, as shown in the example in Figure 3.5. It is best to review the recommended hardware and software requirements before enrolling in an online course. Some of the basic software applications used to complete assignments include word processing, spreadsheet or a database, and presentation programs. Any multimedia plug-ins should be available as free downloads from the Internet. Peripherals, such as a printer and speakers, are usually required as well. A reliable Internet connection, such as a 56K dial-up modem, DSL, or cable, will be needed. It is recommended to have the fastest Internet connection as possible because the instructional files

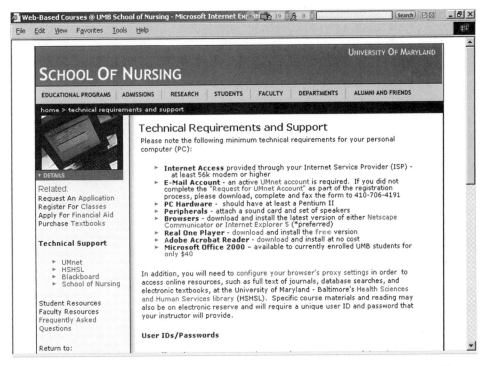

FIGURE 3.5 Screenshot of technical requirements and support. © 2004 University of Maryland School of Nursing.

may contain multimedia content and hence, tend to be huge. Downloading these files over a dial-up connection can be tedious and time consuming. For accessing the courseware management system, a preferred web browser might be recommended. In addition, e-mail accounts are typically provided by the institution and may be the required mechanism for course communication; however, students often can forward incoming e-mails to their own personal e-mail accounts.

In addition to posting information about the course and college online, various methods for informing students about online courses expectations include an orientation letter and e-mails to registered students.

Technical Skills

Students do not need to be computer experts to enroll in an online course. However, they should be comfortable with the following minimum basic computer skills:

- Using a mouse and the concept of a single-click versus a double-click.
- Keyboarding (i.e., typing at least 30 to 40 words per minute).
- Opening and closing software programs.
- Saving and opening files to and from floppy disks or hard drives.

● Copying and/or cutting text and pasting in another location.
● Logging on to the Internet and locating web sites.
● Sending and receiving e-mail.

There are many online tutorials (or checklists) through which students can assess their computer competency. Although technical skills are important, students should also consider if online learning is suited for them depending on their learning styles, commitment, and study habits.

Virtual Orientation and Frequently Asked Questions

Many students will not want to come to campus for an orientation about online coursework. Figure 3.6 shows a screen from an online virtual orientation that contains audio and video narrations and/or animations about e-mail accounts, technical requirements, and using the courseware management system. It even provides testimonials from students who have previously enrolled in online courses.

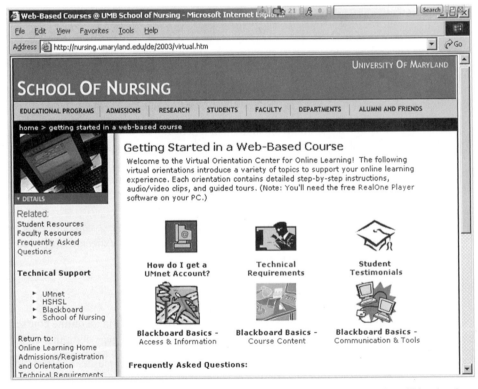

FIGURE 3.6 Screenshot of virtual orientation information. © 2004 University of Maryland School of Nursing.

Providing a Frequently Asked Questions (FAQ) link will greatly reduce the number of questions students will ask the admissions office, registration office, instructors, and technical support staff. The FAQs should include answers to the following questions:

● I registered for an online course. What should I do next?
● I registered for an online course and can log into the courseware management system, but my course doesn't appear. What should I do?
● I already have an e-mail account. Why do I need another one?
● Help! How can I get assistance reviewing the technical requirements?

CONCLUSION

There is no one complete and uniform approach for the technological infrastructure to support for the implementation of web-based distance education. Various approaches have been by employed by campuses to meet their unique environment. This chapter has emphasized the critical success factors that support web-based distance education initiatives—information and instructional technologists, management systems for online delivery of instruction, tools for creating interactive instructional materials, means for accessing scholarly resources, and end-user support. It is important to consider the costs and benefits, as the success of any web-based distance education program ultimately must answer the following question: Will these technology investments lead to improvements in educational quality, effectiveness, and cost reduction?

■ LEARNING ACTIVITIES

● List the advantages and disadvantages of outsourcing technical support and infrastructure delivery mechanisms to an application service provider. What about instructional design?
● Conduct a preliminary analysis of your campus' infrastructure (staff, Internet connectivity, operating systems, server capacity, and multimedia capabilities). What are the strengths and weaknesses? What additional funds and/or resources might be necessary to support online instruction?
● Prepare a presentation describing how technology investments can lead to improvements in educational quality, effectiveness, and cost reduction.

REFERENCES

Association for Educational Communications and Technology (2005). Accreditation standards for programs in educational communications and instructional technology (ECIT). Retrieved August 29, 2005, from http://www.aect.org/standards/history.html
Brace, S. B., & Roberts, G. (1996, March 31–April 2). *Supporting faculty's development and use of instructional technology.* Murfreesboro, TN: Proceedings of the Mid-South Instructional Technology Conference. (ERIC Document Reproduction Service No. ED 400 814).
Gagne, R., & Briggs, L. (1979). *Principles of instructional design.* (2nd ed.) New York: Holt, Rinehart & Winston.
GNU General Public License. Retrieved October 28, 2003, from http://www.gnu.org/copyleft/gpl.html
Hunter, M. (1982). *Mastery teaching.* El Segundo, CA: Instructional Dynamics, Inc.

Leslie, S. (2003, June 8–11). Important characteristics of course management systems: Findings from the Edutools info project. Retrieved December 10, 2003, from http://www.edtechpost.ca/gems/cms_characteristics. htm

Long, P. (2000). Preparing the campus for tomorrow's network. *Educause Leadership Strategies, Volume 1, Preparing your campus for a networked future.* San Francisco: Jossey-Bass Publishers.

McAlister, M. K., Rivera, J., & Hallam S. (2001). Twelve important questions to answer before you offer a web based curriculum. *Online Journal of Distance Learning Administration, 4*(2). Retrieved August 29, 2005, from http://www.westga.edu/~distance/ojdla/summer42/mcalister42.html

Najjar, L. J. (1996). Multimedia information and learning. *Journal of Educational Multimedia and Hypermedia, 5*(2), 129–150.

Newby, T., Stepich, D., Lehman, J., & Russell, J. (2000). *Instructional technology for teaching and learning: Designing instruction, integrating computers, and using media* (2nd ed.). Upper Saddle River, NJ: Prentice Hall.

Olsen, F. (2001). Getting ready for a new generation of course-management systems [Electronic Version]. *Chronicle of Higher Education, 48*(17), A25–A27.

Palloff, R., & Pratt, K. (2001). *The realities of online teaching.* San Francisco, CA: Jossey-Bass.

Wise, M., & Groom, R. (1996). The effect of enriching classroom learning with the systematic employment of multimedia, *Education,* 11(7), 61–69.

Objectives

Upon completion of this chapter, the learner will be able to:

● Describe U.S. copyright law and its application to online education.
● Discuss the elements of fair use and the TEACH Act.
● Use a checklist to determine if use of copyrighted material in the context of digital education conforms to the TEACH Act.

Key Terms

Copyright: A legal right to exclusive publication production, sale, distribution of some work (the expression, not the idea).

Doctrine of Fair Use: A part of the 1976 Copyright Act (17 USC §107) that offers guidance to faculty about the legal use of copyrighted materials without obtaining the copyright holder's permission.

The Technology, Education, and Copyright Harmonization (TEACH) Act: Allows certain copyrighted works to be digitized and placed online for instructional purposes.

CHAPTER FOUR

Legal Considerations

■ ANN MECH AND
BARBARA G. COVINGTON

Chapter Outline

his chapter provides an overview of U.S. copyright law and its application to online education. Copyright ownership of course materials, as well as fair use of copyrighted materials and the TEACH Act, will be discussed. Issues surrounding privacy of student and patient information will be presented in the context of web-based communication. Cyber-cheating is a growing concern in academia. Methods to both prevent and detect it will be outlined.

COPYRIGHT

The federal statute protecting copyright derives its authority from the United States Constitution, Article I, Section 8, Clause 8: "The Congress shall have Power . . . To promote the Progress of Science and useful Arts, by securing for limited Times to Authors and Inventors the exclusive Right to their respective Writings and Discoveries." The Constitution grants Congress the authority to enact laws to provide copyright protection to authors for a time-limited period.

The first copyright statute was enacted in 1790. The copyright law has been substantially revised four times, the most recent major revision in 1976 (17 USC §101, et al.). The 1976 revision of the copyright act provides copyright protections as soon as the author's creative idea is fixed or recorded in a tangible medium of expression. A tangible medium of expression may be words printed on paper, artworks painted on canvas, films and videos, sound recordings, and, most recently, information digitally displayed on the Internet. Basic copyright rights are held by the author even without registration of the work with the Copyright Office. Basic copyright rights for the author include the exclusive right to: make copies of the work; prevent others from making copies of the work; display, perform, and distribute the work; and control any derivative works. A copyright holder may sue to have the infringement of his or her copyright stopped (injunctive relief). If the copyright was registered when the infringement occurred, monetary damages and recovery of attorney fees are available. Copyright protection is secure until 70 years after the death of the author (Miller & Davis, 2000).

Copyright may be held by the author or by anyone to whom the author assigns the copyright, such as to a publisher who will publish and distribute the author's work. An employer may hold copyright rights to employees' work if the work is a "work made for hire" made within the scope of an employee's employment at the direction and under the control of the employer (Miller & Davis, 2000).

An exception to the "work made for hire" rule has been the ownership rights of university faculty in their lectures and course materials. The "Teacher Exception" was established under the 1909 Copyright Act by case law, which cited a long-held tradition that university faculty owned the courses they produced. The "Teacher Exception" was not mentioned in the 1976 Copyright Act. However, a 1987 case from the United States Courts of Appeal for the Seventh Circuit ruled the "Teacher Exception" was now a creation of university policy (Townsend, 2003).

As a result, universities have adopted policies outlining ownership rights in course lectures and other course materials. These policies may separate ownership rights by amount of university resources used to produce the lectures and course materials. If faculty produce lectures and course materials using few university resources (as in the case of live lectures), university policy may allow the faculty to hold ownership rights. In such a case, university policy may state the university has a nonexclusive right to use lectures and course materials otherwise owned by the faculty. That means the university can maintain lectures and course materials even if the faculty–developer leaves university employment.

If, however, there is substantial use of university resources in the production of the course, the university can claim rights to own the course. Online courses often involve substantial use of university resources in their production and certainly in their maintenance. However, even if the university can claim ownership rights in the online course, a faculty–developer may also be able to assert an ownership right in the portion of the course developed by the faculty using little university resources (e.g., faculty produced PowerPoint slides incorporated into the online course). Faculty could then use these slides in other works not controlled by the university. Copyright protects the originality of a work, but originality does not mean exclusivity. A copyrighted work may include components that can be or already have been subject to copyright protection. For example, an article appearing in a scholarly journal with a copyright held by the journal's publisher likely contains referenced content from previously published (and copyrighted) articles. Online courses may be composites of both original and previously copyrighted works. The original portions of the online course may, in turn, be developed by faculty alone or in concert with other university staff using university resources. Thus, determination of ownership rights to online courses is not always straightforward.

Faculty should check university policies to determine the university's position on ownership of online courses and course components, as well as any policies on conflict of interest. This is particularly important if the use of courses or course materials outside of university-sponsored programs is contemplated. A university may restrict distribution of material in which it claims an ownership right, and it may also restrict a faculty's distribution of faculty-owned course material to the university's competitors under its conflict of interest policies.

FAIR USE

Faculty preparing courses and course materials routinely use information that has been previously published and, therefore, copyrighted. They are faced with questions about whether or not the copyrighted material can be incorporated into their courses at all and, if so, if permission from the copyright holder must be obtained. The doctrine of fair use, a part of the Copyright Act (1976), offers guidance to faculty about the legal use of copyrighted materials without obtaining the copyright holder's permission.

The doctrine of fair use allows the use of materials protected by copyright law under certain circumstances without the permission of the copyright holder. Use of copyrighted materials outside of these limited circumstances constitutes copyright infringement. The circumstances constituting fair use were outlined in the 1976 Copyright Act and encompass four areas of analysis:

1. The purpose and character of the use.
2. The nature of the copyrighted work.
3. The proportion of the work that was used.
4. The economic impact of the use.

Consideration of the purpose and character of the use weighs a number of factors. Is the use for commercial or noncommercial endeavors? Is the user a nonprofit or for-profit entity? Is the use for educational programs, literary criticism, or news reporting? How close is the date of use to the date of first publication? Was there sufficient time for the user to obtain the copyright holder's permission to use the work (and pay any required royalty fees)? It may be a fair use for a faculty member to copy and distribute a newspaper article the same day it was first printed. It may not be fair use to copy and distribute it several weeks later or continue to use it in succeeding semesters without obtaining the copyright owner's permission (Miller & Davis, 2000).

Works such as scholarly papers that are expected to be used, referenced, and perhaps quoted by other authors in subsequent publications are a type of copyrighted work for which a fair use may be claimed. The nature of scholarly publications creates a presumption that such publications will be incorporated into future works, albeit appropriately referenced. However, works not created or published with an expectation of subsequent incorporation into future works, such as whole films or musical scores, are not automatically eligible for a claim of fair use (Miller & Davis, 2000).

The amount or proportion of the work used is a factor in determining fair use. There are both quantitative and qualitative measures of proportion. Copying and distributing multiple chapters of a single textbook would not be fair use, even if done for educational purposes. Similarly, copying and distributing key components of a copyrighted work constitute infringement. Key components could be titles and headings, introductions or chapter summaries, or tables and graphs that convey substantial information.

Finally, and most importantly, the economic impact of the use must be weighed. What impact will the use have on the copyright holder's market? For example, one may not claim fair use of a work for educational purposes if the copyright holder's market is in the educational arena. Using a copyrighted work in a manner that diminishes the work's market value could constitute infringement, even if the manner of use might fit into one of the other categories of fair use (Miller & Davis, 2000).

In addition to the four rules of fair use contained in Section 107 of the Copyright Act (1976), Section 110(1) allows teachers in nonprofit educational institutions to display almost any copyrighted work for instructional purposes, including showing a legally obtained videotape in its entirety, during face-to-face classroom teaching. However, the right to display copyrighted works is time-limited: permission of the copyright holder should be obtained if the teacher intends to use copyrighted materials repeatedly in the same class (Harper, 2002a).

Fair Use in the Digital Age

The doctrine of fair use arose in a time of live lectures and paper copies of course hand-outs. Distance and online education came into wide use after the Copyright Act (1976) was enacted. Several aspects of copyright privileges contained in the act make fair use of copyrighted materials in distance and online courses difficult or not feasible.

The fair use doctrine permits the making of copies for distribution under certain circumstances, such as classroom teaching in a nonprofit educational institution. The copies made, however, must be exact replicas of the copyrighted work. Changing the work into a digital format for distribution through distance or online education constitutes the making of a derivative work, which is a right controlled by the copyright holder and is not subject to fair use.

The right of fair use of copyrighted materials in the classroom or similar place devoted to instruction was meant to take place where there was a teacher interacting face-to-face with students in the same room. The students in distance education classes are often located in a classroom many miles from where the teacher is broadcasting. The online classroom is virtual, and teacher and students are separated by not only distance but also time. Finally, students in online courses most likely receive instruction in their homes, not in classrooms or similar places of instruction (Gasaway, 2001).

Section 110(2) of the Copyright Act (1976) permits use of copyrighted materials in distance education classrooms that meet the definitions found in Section 110(1): The class is being conducted under the auspices of a nonprofit educational institution, and the copyrighted work is directly related to the instructional content of the course. The transmission must be received in a classroom or other place normally devoted to instruction or by someone who is prevented by disability from coming to a classroom. As in face-to-face instruction, the use of copyrighted works is time-limited. Permission of the copyright holder is needed if the work is to be transmitted in subsequent semesters. However, Section 110(2) does not permit the transmission of entire dramatic or audiovisual works or complete musical scores. In order to meet fair use restrictions in distance education, only small portions or clips of such works may be transmitted (Diotalevi, 2003; Harper, 2001).

TEACH ACT

At the end of 2002, Congress updated the 1976 Copyright Act to reflect the realities of fair use in teaching in the digital age. The Technology, Education, and Copyright Harmonization (TEACH) Act (2002) allows certain copyrighted works to be digitized and placed online for instructional purposes. However, there are a number of conditions that must be met in order to make online use of copyrighted works not an infringement of the copyright holder's rights.

Although the TEACH Act permits the display of almost all types of works, the display of dramatic and musical works is limited to "reasonable and limited portions." An entire performance (movie, musical score) may not be transmitted. Digitization of analog works is allowed as long as the work is not also produced in digital format, and it contains no technological protections against copying or digitization. Works specifically made for distance or online education, illegally made copies, and works normally purchased by students are not covered by the TEACH Act. The temporary reproduction of a work necessary for the processing of digital transmissions is not considered an infringement. Storage and retention of the copies is allowed, but the time limits of fair use still apply (Bruwelheide, 2003).

As in the earlier version of Section 110(2), the TEACH Act requires the online instruction be part of the educational program of a nonprofit educational institution. There is an additional requirement placed on the educational institution: At the collegiate level, the institution must be accredited by a "regional or national accrediting agency recognized by the Council on Higher Education Accreditation or the U.S. Department of Education." Such institutions must have drafted copyright policies, provide education about copyright, and post notice that works transmitted may be copyright protected (Bruwelheide, 2003).

The online transmission must not only be an integral part of the course; it must also be part of the classroom portion of the course. Online transmission of supplemental readings that are copyright protected, for example, is not permitted through the TEACH Act. The locations eligible to receive transmissions have been expanded beyond classrooms and other sites devoted to instruction to fit today's online student whose computer is in the home (Bruwelheide, 2003).

A checklist to guide faculty in determining if use of copyrighted materials in the context of digital education conforms to the requirements of the TEACH Act has been developed by Georgia Harper, General Counsel for the University of Texas (Box 4.1).

However, it is important for faculty to remember that the TEACH Act does not override the doctrine of fair use. The TEACH Act merely extends the ability to use copyrighted materials beyond the traditional classroom and face-to-face education. The use of copyrighted materials in both traditional and digital classrooms is always subject to the overarching rules of fair use.

OBTAINING PERMISSION TO USE COPYRIGHTED MATERIALS

If the planned use of copyrighted materials does not fall into the safe harbors of the TEACH Act and fair use, permission from the copyright holder must be sought. The copyright holder may or may not be the author of the work. In the case of books or journal articles, the copyright holder likely is the publisher. For musical recordings, it is probably the record label; for movies, the studio or independent producer holds the copyright. There are a number of resources to facilitate identification of the copyright owner and to obtain the owner's permission to use. A list of organizations through which copyright permission may be sought is found in Box 4.2.

Written permission to use copyrighted material is best. If written permission does not come, it is important to document all oral conversations with the copyright holder and send a follow-up letter to the copyright holder confirming any oral discussions and the terms and conditions of any permission to use the work that may have been given. Permission requests should be clear about the intended use of the copyrighted work, especially if there is any intention of use for commercial purposes. The request should also include all possible media for distribution of the work (e.g., web-based, CD-ROM) (Harper, 2003). The user of copyrighted materials does not gain the same rights of ownership the copyright holder

TEACH Act Checklist

BOX 4.1

☐ My institution is a nonprofit accredited educational institution or a governmental agency.

☐ It has a policy on the use of copyrighted materials.

☐ It provides accurate information to faculty, students, and staff about copyright.

☐ Its systems will not interfere with technological controls within the materials I want to use.

☐ The materials I want to use are specifically for students in my class.

☐ Only those students will have access to the materials.

☐ The materials will be provided at my direction during the relevant lesson.

☐ The materials are directly related and of material assistance to my teaching content.

☐ My class is part of the regular offerings of my institution.

☐ I will include a notice that the materials are protected by copyright.

☐ I will use technology that reasonably limits the students' ability to retain or further distribute the materials.

☐ I will make the materials available to the students only for a period of time that is relevant to the context of a class session.

☐ I will store the materials on a secure server and transmit them only as permitted by this law.

☐ I will not make any copies other than the one I need to make the transmission.

☐ The materials are of the proper type and amount the law authorizes:
   Entire performances of nondramatic literary and musical works.
   Reasonable and limited parts of a dramatic literary, musical, or audio-visual works.
   Displays of other works, such as images, in amounts similar to typical displays in face-to-face teaching.

☐ The materials are not among those the law specifically excludes from its coverage:
   Materials specifically marketed for classroom use for digital distance education.
   Copies that are known to be illegal.
   Textbooks, course packs, electronic reserves, and similar materials typically purchased individually by the students for independent review outside the classroom or class session.

☐ If I am using an analog original, I checked before digitizing it to be sure:
   I copied only the amount that I am authorized to transmit.
   There is no digital copy of the work available except with technological protections that prevent my using it for the class in the way the statute authorizes.

Reprinted with permission of Georgia Harper, General Counsel for the University of Texas.

Resources for Obtaining Copyright Permission

Text

- Copyright Clearance Center—http://www.copyright.com
- U.S. Copyright Office—http://www.loc.gov/copyright/

Images

- Academic Press' Image Directory
- American Society of Media Photographers—http://www.asmp.org

Authors

- UnCover
- Publication Rights Clearance House (National Writers Union)—
  http://www.nwu.org

Music

- American Society of Composers, Authors and Publishers—
  http://www. ascap.com
- Broadcast Music, Inc.—http://www.bmi.com
- SESAC—http://www.sesac.com
- Music Research Consultants—http://www.musicresearch.com

Movies

- The Motion Picture Licensing Corporation—http://www.mplc.com

Compiled by Barbara Covington and Diane Fuller of the University of Maryland–Baltimore

possesses. The user may only copy, distribute, or otherwise use the material in accordance with the specifications of the permission granted. What the user gets is a license to use the copyrighted material, and most likely the license is nonexclusive. A nonexclusive license to use the copyrighted material can be given to an unlimited number of users by the copyright holder. This means material such as slides or film clips used in one university course could also be licensed for use by a competing university.

PRIVACY ISSUES IN ONLINE EDUCATION

The Family Educational Rights and Privacy Act (1974), also known as FERPA or the Buckley Amendment, is a federal law regulating the disclosure of student records. Its aim is to protect the privacy of a student's educational records and requires the student's permission (or the permission of a parent if the student is a minor) to disclose educational records beyond the limited number of faculty and staff in the educational institution who need to have such information in the course of their employment.

Faculty should be mindful of the need to protect a student's privacy when communicating student evaluations, grades on coursework, counseling of students, and in other instances where the need to maintain a student's privacy is necessary. The same issues surrounding privacy of student records that is present in face-to-face education exist in online education.

The Health Insurance Portability and Accountability Act (1996), better known as HIPAA, was enacted to protect the privacy of an individual's health information (Protected Health Information or PHI) when transmitted electronically for purposes concerning filing health care claims or coordinating health care benefits. Transmission of health information in an online educational context would not be, by definition, a HIPAA covered transaction. However, state laws governing maintenance of confidentiality of health information still apply to use of that information in any course, whether it is online or face-to-face. Furthermore, if the university, as part of its operations, employs health care providers who treat patients and electronically transmits protected health information in a HIPAA covered transaction, the university may become a covered entity subject to the HIPAA privacy rule. This is often the case at health sciences universities that have faculty-run health care practices. A covered entity must assure compliance with the HIPAA privacy rule controlling dissemination of PHI in any context, not just in electronic claims processing (Standards for Privacy of Individually Identifiable Health Information, 45 CFR 160 and 164). Faculty preparing online courses that incorporate real patient care information in case studies or other teaching tools must adhere to the HIPAA privacy rule regulating disclosure of PHI if the university is a covered entity. Faculty must also comply with state patient confidentiality laws if they are stricter than HIPAA or if HIPAA does not apply.

AMERICANS WITH DISABILITIES ACT AND ONLINE EDUCATION

The Americans with Disabilities Act (1990), otherwise known as the ADA, was enacted to set enforceable standards to eliminate discrimination against individuals with disabilities. Prior to enactment of the ADA, Congress had found that discrimination against individuals with disabilities persisted in employment, housing, transportation, education, communication, and public accommodations. In higher education, the goal of the ADA was to assure access to individuals with disabilities regardless of the college or university's size, nonprofit status, or receipt of federal or public funds. The goal is to provide reasonable and appropriate academic accommodations according to the laws for the students who qualify and who identify themselves. Online education in higher education institutions and post secondary institutions do have ADA and Section 504 of the Rehabilitation Act requirements to meet related to equal access, but other requirements differ for them. The areas that differ are specific to any changes needing to be made to essential elements of the curricula that might compromise the curricular standards. More in-depth information about these differences can be found in *Learning Disabilities: Issues in Higher Education* (National Joint Committee on Learning Disabilities, 2005) or at the U.S. Department of Education web site: http://www.ed.gov.

In online education, the first group of requirements is the infrastructure requirements, which address the student needs related to registration, advising, counseling, and the other parts of the student's life while a student is in a particular program. The second group of requirements is related to the online learning itself.

The infrastructure requirements to support students in the virtual academic setting must be clearly identified in terms of funds, personnel, policies, and procedures and need to be comprehensive in nature, covering from the recruitment phase for the student through registration and advising, to teaching and graduation (National Joint Committee on Learning Disabilities, 2005). By planning for online registration for students, along with phone or mail-in registration, telephone or online advising by faculty, student affairs personnel to assist with financial aid paperwork, and online or mail textbook ordering and other services, the infrastructure requirements will be in place for all students, both traditional and online, and will stand ready to serve those needing accommodations.

The online learning itself is dependent on the student, the faculty, and the institution. Luckily, today there are many hardware and software adaptive devices and software programs available to help online learners and teachers meet ADA requirements. Some of these programs are now standard in desktop computer systems and software packages, which include print enlargers, speech recognition, and phonetic spell checkers. Other adaptive devices, including text-to-speech, reading programs, and textbooks on tape, continue to emerge for higher education (Carlson, 2004; National Joint Committee on Learning Disabilities, 2005).

It is important to remember the needs and appropriate ADA accommodations for students are determined on a case-by-case basis. The institution or faculty is not required to have a crystal ball to see who will be in a class in the future and to build in accommodations for them in the present. But, on the proactive side, if a few points are remembered and addressed in the development phase for an online course, the course will automatically have built into it many of the most common accommodation needs. Courses should be developed with attention given to adult learning, online learning, and instructional design principles. The top principles are as follows:

- Course material is laid out in an organized manner on each screen.
- There is consistency through the course for the navigation guides.
- There is good visual contrast for text, numbers, and images.
- The student is able to select content material presentation options such as visual (videotape lecture), text only, and voice only.

This development approach is also more cost-effective and realistic than waiting to retrofit accommodation needs into an established online course. Even if the course never has one identified student needing accommodations, this course will come closer to meeting the learning needs of our diverse student populations and their many learning styles.

CONCLUSION

The infrastructure required to support students in the academic setting—physical and virtual—needs to be clearly identified in terms of funds, personnel, policies, and procedures. The requirement identification effort must be comprehensive in nature, covering from the recruitment phase for the student through registration and advising, to the teaching and graduation. The laws are complex, but there are many resources available to assist any institution, student, or faculty to understand the laws. Care needs to be taken to understand the laws because they differ to some degree by institution type, disability, and program (National Joint Committee on Learning Disabilities, 2005).

■ LEARNING ACTIVITIES

Read each situation below and apply what you have learned in this chapter to decide if you need to obtain copyright permission to use the item in your online web course. After you have answered the questions, discuss your answers in small groups.

- You have a great journal article from this month you want to post to the discussion board in your web course for each student, this semester only, to read and comment on.
- You want to add a streaming video clip into your web course from a CD-ROM you bought at a conference.
- You have great student pictures you want to add into your course to demonstrate how much fun online learning can be.
- You have some clinical pictures of patients you want to include in your course modules on the web, and you have permissions for the hardcopy photographs to be used for teaching purposes.
- You have a book that is no longer in publication and want to scan in the book pages for your students to read as part of your online course. The author is deceased, and the book is not being advertised online for sale even as a used or old book.

REFERENCES

Americans with Disabilities Act, 42 USC §12101 (1990).

Bruwelheide, J. (2003). TEACH Act highlights and resources. Retrieved November 16, 2003 from http://nea.org/he/abouthe/teachact.html

Carlson, S. (2004, June 11). Left out online. *The Chronicle of Higher Education,* 50(40), A23–A25. Retrieved September 20, 2005 from http:///chronicle.com/free/USO/i40/40a 02301.ktm

Copyright Act, 17 USC §101 (1976).

Diotalevi, R. (2003, Winter). An education in copyright law: A primer for cyberspace. *Electronic Journal of Academic and Special Librarianship, 4*(1), Retrieved April 29, 2004 from http://nea.org/he/abouthe/teachact.html

Family Educational Rights and Privacy Act, 20 USC §31.1232g (1974).

Gasaway, L. (2001). Balancing copyright concerns: The TEACH Act of 2001. *EDUCAUSE review,* Nov/Dec 2001, 82–83.

Harper, G. (2001). Educational fair use guidelines for distance learning. Retrieved November 24, 2003 from http://utsystem.edu/ogc/intellectualproperty/distguid.htm

Harper, G. (2002a). Fair use of copyrighted materials. November 24, 2003 from http://utsystem.edu/ogc/intellectualproperty/copypol2.htm

Harper, G. (2002b). The TEACH Act finally becomes law. Retrieved October 16, 2003 from http://utsystem.edu/ocg/intellectualproperty/teachact.htm

Harper, G. (2003). Getting permission. Retrieved October 23, 2003 from http://utsystem.edu/ogc/intellectualproperty

Health Insurance Portability and Accountability Act, 42 USC §7.1320d–1320–8 (1996).

Miller, M., & Davis, A. (2000). *Intellectual property: Patents, trademarks and copyright* (3rd ed.). St. Paul, MN: West Group.

National Joint Committee on Learning Disabilities. (2005) Learning disabilities: Issues in higher education. Austin, TX: Pro-Ed Publications. Retrieved January 22, 2005 from http://www.idonline.org/njcld/higher_ed.html

Standards for Privacy of Individually Identifiable Health Information, 45 CFR Parts 160 and 164.

Townsend, E. (2003). Legal and policy responses to the disappearing "teacher exception" or copyright ownership in the 21st century university. *4 Minn. Intell. Prop. Rev.209.* Retrieved September 13, 2005 from http://mipr.umn.edu/archive/v4n2/townsend.pdf

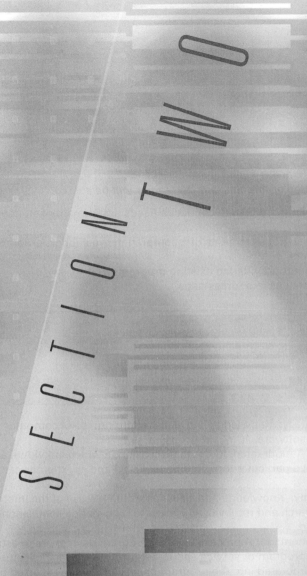

SECTION TWO

Development
of a Virtual
Learning
Community

Objectives

Upon completion of this chapter, the learner will be able to:

- Create a preliminary plan to conduct a needs assessment of student support requirements.
- Describe the various elements of a comprehensive support program for online learners.
- Analyze support provided in existing programs.
- Develop strategies to address gaps.

Key Terms

Computer Literacy: Knowledge and skills regarding use of computer hardware and software.

Focus Group: A moderated, in-depth discussion in which individual and group opinions about a particular topic can be explored and key themes can be identified.

Internet Literacy: Knowledge and skills regarding the use of the Internet for information search and retrieval, as well as for knowledge acquisition and communication.

Needs Assessment: (a) A process used by program developers to establish the need for a program or service and to determine the specific features that should be incorporated into the program or service; (b) the reported outcome of the process of assessing need.

Stakeholders: The individuals or groups who have a vested interest in the outcomes of a program.

Student Support: The information, resources, coaching, protocols and/or processes provided to students to promote effective and satisfactory online learning.

System User Interface: The juncture between the users of online programs and the technology that allows them to access the software, hardware, and courseware for the program.

Virtual Orientation: The process of orienting students to the software, hardware, and courseware required for a specific online offering (course or program); orientation focuses upon technological and user knowledge, skills and development of favorable attitudes, and perceived self-efficacy regarding online learning.

CHAPTER FIVE

Creating a Supportive Environment for Online Learning

■ NALINI JAIRATH

Chapter Outline

*S*tudent support, or the creation of a learning environment that meets the perceived needs of students, is an essential consideration in crafting effective online educational programs and courses. The use of the word *student* in this chapter reflects the recognition that provision of support is essentially a consumer service activity in which meeting the requirements of individuals who assume the student role is paramount. Student support has been identified as a major indicator of the quality of online educational offerings (Institute for Higher Education Policy, 2000). Inadequate support may be related to lowered student satisfaction with the quality of online education, poorer educational outcomes, and lower completion rates for courses and programs. Student support involves the provision to students of information, resources, coaching, protocols and/or processes that enhance the quality of the learning environment (Forman, Nyatanga, & Rich, 2002; Institute for Higher Education Policy, 2000; Oehlkers & Gibson, 2001).

The responsibility for student support is assumed by the faculty, the technological staff, and the academic program. More explicitly, the purpose of student support is to:

- Prevent technological problems from adversely impacting the quality of online education received by students.
- Maximize the unique benefits or added value of online relative to traditional educational offerings.
- Support student perceptions of a helpful, responsive learning environment.

Based on this description and the associated purposes, student support is not an all-or-nothing phenomenon; rather, it ranges along a continuum of quality. The upper end of the continuum is the provision of support that is cost-effective, time-efficient, rapid, responsive, and tailored to specific student needs. Student support requires a systematic, comprehensive approach that is integrated into planning and implementation activities for online education and for traditional education with online enhancement. Other chapters have addressed student support within the context of developing an infrastructure for online learning, clinical teaching, and course development. Therefore, this chapter focuses upon the use of program planning approaches for program development and the key elements of student support programs.

NEEDS ASSESSMENT AS THE BASIS OF PROGRAM PLANNING

This chapter addresses the way in which a student support program tailored to the needs of the individual online educational program can be developed. The approach described is based on general principles and approaches to program development in the health sciences, such as those most recently described by Issel (2004). The basis of program planning is clear identification of student support requirements and of the situational factors that influence the ability to meet these requirements. Needs assessments may be used to obtain this information. The term *needs assessment* is used in two ways: (a) to describe the process used to establish need, as in "a needs assessment established that . . ."; or (b) to describe the findings of an assessment, as in "the needs assessment supported the

Purposes of Needs Assessments

Exploration: to obtain information regarding the feasibility of establishing an online program or course.

Decision making: to determine the benefits versus the drawbacks of using web-enhancement or converting a traditional course or program to an online offering.

Resource allocation: to determine the resources that need to be allocated after the decision has been made about an online program or course.

Evaluation: to routinely examine the adequacy of existing resources after a program or course or when concerns exist about student support.

importance of. . . ." For the purposes of this chapter, both approaches are used; in general, however, a needs assessment of student support requirements consists of information gathered in advance of a program that documents the demand for the program and the program features that are desired by the user. Box 5.1 provides a general overview of the purposes of needs assessment. The needs assessment permits the individuals responsible for online education to determine student support requirements as well as the available resources to meet these needs. To ensure that the needs assessment is comprehensive, faculty, instructional media specialists and/or personnel, and those responsible for the technological infrastructure should all participate. A systematic approach should be used to conduct the needs assessment. The process of conducting a needs assessment involves planning, implementing, analyzing, and evaluating needs assessment data.

PLANNING AND IMPLEMENTING THE NEEDS ASSESSMENT

Planning the needs assessment requires careful thought and attention to detail. The process of planning is presented as a series of sequential activities to help the reader understand what is involved; however, in practice, these activities are rarely completed in a step-by-step manner; instead, the individuals planning the needs assessment may go back and forth as new considerations are determined.

Identification of the Purpose of the Assessment

An additional consideration is to determine whether the assessment pertains to a particular course or to an entire program. The exact focus and scope of the needs assessment is shaped by the time frame of the overall online project, the projected uses of the data, and the resultant decisions. In structuring the needs assessment, it is helpful to establish whether the assessment is for use by the organization alone or whether it may conceivably be incorporated into current and future grant-related activities and to justify additional program growth in the future. This distinction is especially important for online programs that are projected to increase in scope or when discrete online courses are offered as a prelude to offering an entire academic program online. For example, needs assessment data that indicated strong program capability to meet student support requirements may be used to justify the growth of new online programs or development of off-shoots of existing programs. In general, when the data have additional value beyond their original purpose, it may be helpful to use a more rigorous approach analogous to that used to conduct a research study. For example, it may be reasonable to pay greater attention to the validity and reliability of data collected and data collection approaches.

Identification of Methods and Procedures

Once the purpose of the needs assessment has been determined, the methods and procedures involved in conducting the needs assessment (i.e., the methodology), are determined. The activities involved in identifying the methodology for the needs assessment are adapted from those used in program evaluation and in research (Issel, 2004). They include sampling, design, and data collection procedures.

Sampling

Sampling refers to the way in which participants in the needs assessment are selected. Usually, sampling is not confined to one group alone; rather, all stakeholders are included, although their relative importance may vary. The concept of *stakeholders* is important for those planning a needs assessment to understand. Stakeholders may simply be understood as individuals or groups who have a vested interest in the success of the on-line offering. Thus stakeholders include students (i.e., users), the organization sponsoring the offering, administrators, faculty, and information technology (IT) personnel. Students are stakeholders as the users of support services; if support is inadequate, students' ability to complete online programs successfully is jeopardized. The organization and administrators are stakeholders because adequate student support is critical to the educational mission. IT personnel are stakeholders because they may be assigned major responsibilities for providing online support. Faculty are stakeholders because their responsibilities for student support increase as the adequacy of other support procedures decrease. For example, if students receive inadequate orientation to online offerings, they may require more coaching from faculty.

Once the stakeholders have been identified, the needs assessment team should choose a sampling approach to determine the number and features of stakeholders in each category from whom needs assessment data should be collected. The goal of sample selection is to ensure that the sample is representative of the larger group of stakeholders. The number of individuals sampled may vary depending upon the scope of the needs assessment. The sampling approach is most important when considering student stakeholders. It is advisable that the student sample be large enough that the data reflect the needs of the student body and diverse enough that the range of student needs is represented. Thus, sampling is purposeful with the goal of identifying the support needs of students who are novices to online education. Table 5.1 illustrates sample stakeholders for a needs assessment examining student support requirements for a registered nurse to baccalaureate degree (RN to BSN) completion program.

Sample Stakeholders in an RN to BSN Completion Program

TABLE 5.1

STAKEHOLDERS	DATA PROVIDED
Director of the RN to BSN completion program	The degree to which administration is committed to and has the resources to assume student support costs
Faculty teaching both clinical and nonclinical courses	Perspectives regarding the student support issues about which students approach them The relationship between quality of online courses compared to traditional courses
Instructional media specialists and technologists	Technological issues that students need assistance handling Support capabilities of the existing infrastructure
Students who intend to complete their degrees online	Exposure to online education Perceived support needs Competing professional and personal responsibilities that limit their time commitment to their program

Design

Once the sample has been identified, the design for the needs assessment is considered. The term *design* really means the approach to collecting data. Usually a design in which multiple methods are used to collect data will yield the most helpful information because the drawbacks or limitations of any one approach can be compensated for. Methods used include focus groups, surveys or questionnaires, and interviews with key stakeholders. Analysis of existing data from such services as the help desk or existing e-mail communication documenting student questions should also be considered. Although selection of the design and data collection procedures are discussed separately in this chapter, the two activities really occur concurrently and influence each other. Major designs useful for needs assessment of student support are now discussed.

Data Collection
Focus Groups

Focus group methodology for needs assessment and program planning in the health sciences has been addressed extensively (Krueger & Casey, 2000; Mansell, Bennett, Northway, Mead, & Moseley, 2004; McLafferty, 2004). Based on the literature, a focus group consists of a group of individuals who are invited to meet for at least one 60-minute to 90-minute session to discuss a specific topic. Focus group participants may be selected to ensure that a wide variety of opinions about the topic can be determined. Thus, in a focus group examining student support requirements, it may be helpful to include novice users of online education as well as experienced users. Focus group conversation is guided by a moderator or facilitator who uses general questions and probes to explore the topic of interest. The moderator also ensures that the focus group conversation remains true to its purpose and that all participants are able to express their opinions. The focus group allows new or emerging issues related to support needs to be determined. For example, if a participant mentions that viruses affect the ability to use the operating system or courseware, the moderator can move the conversation to an exploration of that theme. Focus groups are typically audiotaped or videotaped, and after the group session is completed, the focus group conversation is analyzed to determine key themes. The analysis takes time and it is customary to reconvene the focus group on a different date to verify or validate that the themes identified accurately capture the opinions of the focus group participants.

Thus, the focus group approach increases the richness of the data or information gathered in the needs assessment. However, the traditional focus group approach has limitations. The focus group requires a skilled moderator who can ensure that the perspectives of all participants are addressed and no participant dominates the discussion. Otherwise, the content of focus group data may be skewed so that it may not provide a clear picture of the frequency of particular student support needs or even of the most important needs. For example, a focus group involving student users could focus on one major topic, such as the need for support with exam taking, and neglect other topics, such as the impact of connectivity issues on access to course information. Analysis of focus group data may be time-consuming, and typically, focus group participants are compensated for their time. Although the traditional focus group approach involves face-to-face contact, the data may not be representative of the student group if geographically distant students are unable to participate because of travel restrictions. One option is to conduct an online focus group, recognizing that some contextual cues associated with face-to-face communication may be missed. Another alternative is to use other data collection approaches, including surveys and questionnaires, interviews, and data from existing databases or data sources.

Surveys and Questionnaires

Surveys and questionnaires address some of the limitations of focus group approaches to collecting data. Surveys and questionnaires can contain close-ended items in which the participant has a fixed set of options from which to choose, or they may have open-ended elements in which the participant is free to write comments. They are relatively easy to administer via phone, mail, or the Internet, and the participant may preserve his or her anonymity. They also allow information that is semi-quantitative to be collected and analyzed. For example, information about the frequency with which participants experience particular support problems could be determined or the degree to which a particular support service is important could be rated.

Despite their benefits, surveys and questionnaires also have limitations. The response rate, that is, the percentage of surveys and questionnaires returned or completed, may limit the ability to apply findings to the larger group of students requiring support. Surveys and questionnaires must also be properly structured so that they provide reliable and valid information. Reliability refers to the ability of the survey or questionnaire to yield the same information when administered either using different methods (i.e., using mail versus Internet) or different administrators (i.e., using different interviewers for phone administration). Reliability may also be of concern if the survey or questionnaire is administered over a period of time during which other events may influence responses.

Validity refers to the ability of the survey or instrument to measure the concept or idea that is being examined. For example, measuring connectivity by asking only whether or not participants have broadband access will not yield a valid measure of connectivity.

Interviews

Interviews represent the third major approach to collecting data for the needs assessment of student support. They may be especially useful when data from stakeholders other than students or faculty are elicited. These other stakeholders include system administrators, academic deans, or department chairs offering online courses. For these nonstudent stakeholders, there may be insufficient numbers for focus groups, and survey or questionnaire construction may be too labor-intensive for the small number of nonstudent stakeholders. In addition, interviews allow extensive exploration and questioning to elicit rich or detailed data. The yield from an interview is strengthened if an interview guide with questions and prompts is developed beforehand.

Existing Data and Databases

In addition to designs in which data are collected directly from stakeholders, analysis of existing data regarding usage patterns of current online program users may yield important information. These data may consist of cached or back-up data documenting Internet usage for a time period. Alternately, it may be data from archived courses, e-mail correspondence with faculty, help service or help desks. These data are especially valuable for understanding the student support requirements arising from the technology-user interface. For example, in some institutions, all routine updating, servicing, and technological modifications occur on weekends or at midnight. The impact of these procedures on student ability to access the system may not be evident until cached data regarding the pattern of student attempts to log on are examined or until stored student discussion board data are examined.

COLLECTING NEEDS ASSESSMENT DATA

Once the general design has been selected, the data to be collected should be specified. In this step, the general objectives are broken down into a series of more concrete questions; the information source and data collection method may then be addressed. The data to be collected will depend on the scope of the needs assessment. In this section, some common data are presented.

Technology Support Assessment Data

Assessment of the support for the technology required for online education should focus on the degree to which the technological infrastructure articulates with the student user's hardware and software and on the interface problems that significantly impact user satisfaction with the online offering. The author's experience and the benchmarks identified as quality indicators for online education (Institute for Higher Education Policy, 2004) suggest that the following questions may be important to ask when technological support is assessed.

How compatible are the registration, fiscal, course delivery, and test administration systems? This question is important to answer because failure of the systems to communicate may adversely affect the quality of the online experience. Without proper articulation, students may have difficulty enrolling in courses, accessing protected course materials, and taking online exams or tests.

What is the impact on the system-to-user interface of student noncompliance with recommendations regarding hardware, operating system, other software, browser setting, and Internet service provider characteristics? Online education has an inherent expense. Students may seek to reduce the expense by using personal computers that lack adequate processing speeds and sufficient random access memory (RAM). They may use modems with low bit rates when broadband is required or older operating systems that do not have the same features as the newer recommended operating systems.

Conversely, upgrades and alternate software used by some students may also adversely affect the system–user interface. Some newer operating systems may lack backward compatibility with courseware. Antiviral software and firewall programs may limit functionality unless customized configurations are used. The net result of one or more of these system–user mismatches may include slow download times, system crashes, jerky streaming of video clips, and blocking of necessary pop-ups.

What are the frequency and nature of problems associated with logging in to courseware? Inability to access courseware in a timely fashion is a major source of dissatisfaction, especially for students who may have to fit online coursework into an already busy schedule. Logging-on problems may arise from several factors, including (a) connectivity issues associated with Internet service providers; (b) security problems associated with password expiration, viruses, and firewalls; and (c) connectivity problems associated with the technological infrastructure. The connectivity problems arising from the infrastructure may reflect the hardware limitations. For dial-up or DSL connections, sample hardware limitations include problems with telephone service, wiring, and lines; for cable connections, sample problems include problems with routers, cable modems, and wiring. Conversely, connectivity problems may reflect scheduling problems. For example, system administrators may choose to load system upgrades on weekends or during the night. However, the around-the-clock nature of online education is such that usage may actually be lower on weekdays than at other times. In examining connectivity problems, the frequency and duration of lost connectivity related to hardware problems should be determined. For scheduling problems, the patterns of user activity should be determined, areas of conflict between high-use times and planned loss of connectivity investigated, and the adequacy of procedures to notify students of the date and time of scheduled updates and resultant downtimes evaluated.

How have technological factors affected students' ability to take online tests and exams? Students find tests and exams stressful at the best of times. Good technological support for online testing is essential. The exact support provided depends on the way that testing has been structured by the faculty member. Technological problems for which students may require support include inability to gain secured access to tests or exams, loss of information during testing due to computer crashes or problems saving responses, and premature closing of exams. This last problem may occur for exams that are timed or for exams that can only be taken within a certain block of time.

Student Characteristics and Behaviors

Based on recent literature (Ali, Hodson-Carlton, & Ryan, 2004; Mosbaek, 1999; Thiele, 2003), the second area that should be explored as part of the needs assessment is the impact of student characteristics and behaviors on support requirements. Based on the author's experiences, the following basic questions should be included in the needs assessment.

What factors motivate students to pursue online education? Although the literature is limited, the author's experience suggests that motivation may be an important factor affecting student satisfaction with online education and the need for support. Factors motivating students to enroll online include the convenience and ease of access to course materials, and compatibility with lifestyle requirements. In contrast, our experience suggests that if students enroll in online courses because no alternative is perceived to exist, student support needs may increase. These students may feel trapped, helpless, and resentful when they encounter technical problems or difficulties related to the online nature of the course.

What are the technological capabilities of students? In general, students who have had prior experience with online education may adapt to new offerings more easily. They are already familiar with such basic activities as logging on, using some form of chat, whether synchronous or asynchronous, and accessing course materials. In contrast, students who have never taken an online course need much more extensive support because they lack a context for online education. The needs of the novice online student can be understood by considering computer literacy and Internet literacy. Computer literacy refers to an individual's degree of basic knowledge regarding basic aspects of personal computing, while Internet literacy refers to an individual's basic understanding of the structure, features, and limitations of the Internet. Both types of literacy range along a continuum with varying degrees of proficiency. The author's experience suggests that computer literacy and Internet literacy affect students' comfort with the technology required for Internet learning. They may also affect students' comfort level in acknowledging support needs as well their ability to describe the problems they encounter in a way that can be understood by those providing technological support. Finally, they may affect students' willingness to try various troubleshooting strategies should technological problems occur.

What is the nature of students' prior experience with online education and the current courseware? Courseware literacy is a term the author has coined to express the student's knowledge and skills regarding courseware used in an online course or program. Courseware literacy is a consideration with both novice and experienced users of online education because popular educational courseware programs such as Angel, Blackboard, and WebCT have different formats. Courseware literacy is essential to derive full benefit from online learning. Students who do not know such basics as where assignments and due dates are posted or how to post messages in chat rooms are severely disadvantaged in an online environment.

What are student courseware utilization patterns? The courseware utilization pattern describes the way in which students use the courseware; utilization may be characterized in terms of the frequency of logging on, the sites in the course visited and the course activities in which students participate, and the total time spent online and its distribution over the duration of the course. Many courseware programs have some internal monitoring capabilities for both individual users and the class as an aggregate such that utilization data are relatively easy to determine. In general, support requirements peak during student orientation to the course, prior to assignments, and when exams or tests are scheduled. These times thus represent periods of high demand for support service. Analysis of utilization patterns can also help identify additional periods when support needs are high, the types of courseware activities that require support, and the period (i.e., day, evening, or night) when courseware use peaks.

How do students meet their online educational support needs? Students have various types of support needs when they take online courses. Our experience suggests that students require both social support and technical support. In the online context, we use social support to indicate students' need to know and to be known by the faculty teaching the course; technical support indicates the students' need for an answer or a solution to a particular problem. Although both methods of support can be provided online, students, especially novice users, may find traditional ways of communication such as phone calls, appointments, or drop-in visits more meaningful than online communication. In contrast, students may post their technical support needs on course bulletin boards, in chat rooms, or e-mail designated help addresses. Technical support needs can usually be addressed via e-mail or phone communication.

Student Support Services

The last major area that should be addressed during data collection for the needs assessment focuses upon the existing student support service. In assessing the adequacy of student support service, both the preventive measures taken to avoid problems and the measures to deal with problems should be addressed. The following questions may be helpful in assessing support service.

What is the nature of student orientation? Appropriate orientation of students to the online learning environment and to the online course is a key preventive step in decreasing student support needs. In assessing the nature of the orientation, it may be helpful to determine:

● The method used to provide the orientation (online or face-to-face).
● Video versus text method of orientation.
● Whether the orientation is mandatory or optional.
● The scope of orientation and student access to orientation material after the orientation period is over.

How do students access help services, and what form of student support services exist? These questions provide information about communication approaches used to seek and provide support. The needs assessment should provide information regarding the existence and use of designated e-mail mailbox, discussion boards addressing technological issues, and help desks or lines. E-mail communication to faculty, postings on discussion boards, and e-mail/phone communication with help desks should also be examined to determine problems with service support approaches. To answer this question, the needs assessment should also address triage services and support for common, potentially severe problems such as those associated with Internet viruses and worms.

What policies and protocols exist to address student service requirements? The vast majority of student support needs that cannot be directly addressed by course faculty pertain to technological difficulties. Therefore, it is essential that policies and protocols exist regarding student service requirements. For example, the needs assessment should address whether policies exist to address computer problems that affect the students' ability to take online tests, and whether a procedure to respond to helping students reschedule tests exists.

What service standards are in place to ensure adequacy of student support? This question addresses the indicators used by the online offering to determine satisfactory responses to student support needs. First, it is necessary to establish whether standards are in place and then to compare data regarding the current support provided to the standards. For example, the needs assessment should compare the average and desired response times to student help requests. Data regarding the average number of encounters with the student until the support need is resolved should also be collected. In addition to examining standards, it is important to determine whether the stakeholders agree about the standards. For example, a 24-hour response time may be viewed as acceptable to program administrators and faculty but may be unacceptable to students.

What institutional and/or administrative support exists for provision of support services? This question really addresses the resource base available to develop and provide student support. The needs assessment should obtain data regarding the current cost and resources used to provide support as well as the projected institutional support. For example, if no dedicated IT personnel exist to provide support, administrative commitment to quality student support is likely to be minimal. Similarly, if IT personnel do not have empathy for the needs of students who have difficulties with the technological aspects of online education, the utilization of IT support by students and their perceptions of IT helpfulness may be low.

ANALYZING NEEDS ASSESSMENT DATA

Once the needs assessment has been conducted and data collected, the data are analyzed to determine an action plan. In general, data analysis is structured about the data collection categories. If a formal report is required, the description of findings and the data analysis approach should be more rigorous and extensive. Data analysis should address each of the broad categories identified in the previous section. The analysis should describe the current support services, the gaps in provision of services, student and other stakeholder satisfaction with current services, and overall administrative commitment. For each of these general categories, the needs assessment should permit at least a narrative description. It is helpful to summarize the key themes or issues that summarize the data for each category. Examples of problems and exemplars of quality are also helpful. In addition to the narrative description presented, basic frequency data are recommended. These data should be presented in such a way that it can be compared to subsequent data for benchmarking. Thus the use of bar graphs or pie charts may be helpful to underscore main findings regarding data analysis. Box 5.2 presents a case study extrapolated from the author's own experiences to illustrate the way in which data from a needs analysis was used to address a problem with student support.

Brief Case Analysis of Inadequate Support for Online Registration

BOX 5.2

Background

A faculty member teaching an online course for the first time found that students were e-mailing her that they could not access the course despite their attempts to enroll. It was taking 1 to 2 weeks to resolve the problem and they were missing class content.

Support Problem

Some students were effectively shut out of the course; this affected their ability to progress in the course and their contribution to the course discussions.

Description of Contributory Factors

The courseware restricted course access to users who were allowed to take online courses and further restricted access to those users enrolled in particular courses. Therefore, the Registrar's Office sent lists of course registrants to the Instructional Media Specialist who then uploaded registrants in a batch so that they could be first recognized as users permitted to have access to online courses; they were then identified as having user status for the particular courses in which they were registered. Some potential users, however, had a financial hold or restriction on their ability to register. In many cases, the hold arose because the tuition support that they received from their employers was delayed. These individuals could thus not be registered in the course unless the faculty member specifically enrolled them in the course. The faculty member was reluctant to do so because she had no way of knowing when the financial issues were resolved.

The faculty member determined that the lag time associated with sorting out these issues was more problematic for online courses. In traditional sections of the course, the student could be given permission by the faculty member to sit in on classes without having to register the student in the course. With online sections that required a student log in and password, this option was not possible.

The faculty member also noted that students developed a contingency plan in which they sometimes shared each others' log ins and passwords so that they would not fall behind in their work. This strategy helped students but resulted in a faculty workload based on an underestimation of course size. It also affected the quality of student participation in the class. From the faculty member's perspective, the magnitude of the student registration problem was underestimated.

Analysis

The Registrar's Office had passed on the major responsibility for the online portion of registration to the Instructional Media Specialist with the faculty member serving as the second individual responsible for identifying students as users. This strategy decreased the workload in the Registrar's Office and avoided the need to provide their staff with the training required for registration of online users. However, it generated a large amount of work for the Instructional Media Specialist who was responsible for 15 to 20 courses each semester. It also generated additional work for faculty and was a cause of considerable stress for students caught in the middle. This approach was in-effective and inappropriate.

Solution

Because this was an issue in other online courses, the faculty member brought the issue before the committee responsible for online education. The institu-tion developed an alternate registration approach in which students with finan-cial holds and other legitimate registration issues were permitted to enroll in the course with an audit status designation. The staff of the Registrar's Office received training in the enrollment management aspects of the online course-ware. The next semester, the Registrar's Office assumed responsibility for updating registration lists and ensuring that the audit designation was converted to regular registration in a timely fashion.

DEVELOPING A STUDENT SUPPORT PROGRAM

Once a comprehensive needs assessment has been conducted and data have been ana-lyzed, a student support program tailored to the individual online offering or program can be developed. Based on the Melbourne Model proposed by Chambers (2004), a student support program should provide support for the stages through which students progress as part of their online education. These stages include recruitment, enrollment, induction, participation, and end with the stage of graduation and beyond. To adequately provide support, the author's experience supplemented by the literature (Chambers, 2004; Insti-tute for Higher Education Policy, 2004) suggests that, at a minimum, student support programs should also address certain essential elements:

● Orientation
● Creation of a learning community
● Technological support

Orientation

The first essential element is an effective orientation program. Orientation may be delivered online, virtually, via CD-ROM, or face-to-face. The online orientation has distinct benefits. It is accessible to those who cannot attend face-to-face orientations because of distance or scheduling concerns. It may also decrease the length of ori-entation for students who already have some familiarity with online learning. Finally, online orientation may be used to model the way in which online learning occurs, and thus may help potential students determine whether online learning is a modality they wish to pursue. The student should be able to complete the online or virtual orientation without needing to log onto the courseware. In some institutions, the virtual orientation is found via a link on the institution's main web page or the web page summarizing online offerings. The virtual orientation may use multiple approaches to orienting the user, including screen shots of various aspects of the courseware, video clips, written information, and slide shows with narrated voice-overs. It is helpful if the virtual orientation is layered, such that more experienced users may skip the content with which they are familiar. Use of CD-ROM technology is of value when potential students may have limited access to the online environment. For example, in rural areas, students may need to travel to a community center or library to access the Internet. Face-to-face orientations may be helpful for novice users who may benefit from the additional coaching.

Regardless of the delivery method, the orientation should include core content regarding the courseware (i.e., the software package or program used to access the course), the way in which the course components are presented using the courseware, and methods of online communication. For example, the orientation should teach the student user how to log on and use courseware main pages. The student should then be introduced to the courseware section containing the course syllabus, course assignments, and such. The student should learn how to communicate with faculty and classmates using such venues as the discussion boards and synchronous and asynchronous chat rooms. The orientation should also introduce the student to the online evaluation approaches with the recognition that more detailed explanation of the methods of online testing should occur in closer proximity to the test dates. The orientation should contain hands-on learning activities to increase student comfort and skills with online learning and allow them to acquire some minimal initial competence in participating in the course.

The second major component of the orientation should address faculty expectations of student behavior and course etiquette. Students should understand the frequency with which they are expected to access course materials, appropriate methods of communicating concerns, appropriate methods of discussing course content, and strategies for working in groups online. They should be reminded that e-mail communication about the course and information posted in chat rooms is not confidential and that they should express themselves appropriately; they should be made aware that course faculty have access to all communication in a course, including group chat rooms.

The third component of the orientation should address strategies for dealing with technological problems. Students should be apprised of the turnaround time for help desks to respond, the e-mail addresses and phone numbers for technological help, and strategies for dealing with technological problems on weekends and outside of business hours.

Finally, the orientation should affirm the positive benefits of online education, the faculty commitment to helping the student enjoy the online course, and the array of support services to assist students.

Creation of a Learning Community

A vital element of student support is creating the perception of being a member of a learning community as opposed to learning in isolation (Palloff & Pratt, 1999). Various strategies exist to create the learning community. These include ensuring that students introduce each other and structuring group activities and projects so that students work together. Use of video clips of students, Web cameras to enhance the online experience, and establishment of times for synchronous communication are all helpful. The learning community is also enhanced by the quality of the faculty support. Faculty must participate in the course frequently and should also use e-mail and phone communication to draw more isolated students into the community.

Technological Support

Technological problems are a major issue affecting student satisfaction with online education and may represent a major gap in the quality of student support. Technology support requirements may be considered in terms of the type of technological problems that can be addressed and the way in which the user and technology staff communicate and work together. Because technological problems affecting functioning of courseware may originate from external factors such as viruses or loss of connectivity, the technology support provided to students must have diagnostic capabilities. It may be useful to offer compatible anti-spyware, antiviral, and firewall programs, operating systems, and personal computers at an educationally discounted rate. This strategy may help ensure that the courseware runs appropriately.

The communication process is equally challenging and it is recommended that the process of technology support include four features. First, each course should have a discussion board section where students can post questions and receive answers about common difficulties; this discussion board should be checked daily by the IT support staff. Second, courseware main pages should have a section or link to frequently asked questions (FAQs) about technology. These FAQs may help provide the user with basic information about ways to obtain help and troubleshoot problems. Third, students should be aware of an e-mail address to which questions can be sent. The e-mail inbox should be checked at least daily, usually more frequently. An automatic message indicating that the e-mail has been received and that the student will receive a reply within 24 hours or less should be generated. Fourth, a log of e-mails should be maintained and frequent problems identified. A standard response to these problems should be generated and when this standard response is used, the student's name should be identified in reply. This transforms the information from a generic message to a personalized response.

The following example indicates how these features work together. A student may find that he or she is unable to log on to the course. A standard reason for this problem is an expired password. With a well articulated technology support system, the student should be able to find the common explanation in the orientation and the FAQs links. If the student sends an e-mail, the student should receive a reply acknowledging the e-mail and the maximum turnaround time within a few minutes. The IT staff will then investigate the problem, and if an expired password is the explanation, address an individualized e-mail containing standard instructions for password renewal.

CONCLUSION

Student support not only includes provision of technological support but also recognition that online learning represents a marked departure from traditional learning approaches. In this chapter, student support has been addressed in terms of a distinct program that should accompany online courses or online programs. Because of this premise, the process of assessing student support requirements and developing a planned program has been a major focus. Finally, essential elements of a student support program have been described.

■ LEARNING ACTIVITIES

- Develop a frequently asked questions (FAQs) guide for an online health science course. Your guide should address at least five FAQs and contain the nontechnological information that a newly enrolled student would need. Describe how the FAQ page might differ for a clinical course as compared to a seminar style course. Discuss the considerations in determining where to position your FAQ guide.
- Interview faculty who are teaching an online course and at least three students who have taken online courses. Identify the common technological problems they have encountered. Develop a standardized e-mail response for each of these problems.
- Compare and contrast the information and coaching approaches used for virtual and face-to-face student orientations to an online educational program.
- You are a faculty member assigned to work with an instructional media specialist to develop an online physical assessment course. Part of your responsibility is to determine student support needs for this course. Develop a guide for a face-to-face versus an online focus group held to determine the support needs that students identify.
- Conduct an Internet search to identify the ways used by health science programs to orient new students to their online educational offerings. Examine at least three programs. Compare and contrast the ways in which each program addresses (a) technological requirements, (b) strategies that students may use to maximize online learning, and (c) the ways in which expected student behaviors and online etiquette are addressed.

REFERENCES

Ali, N. S., Hodson-Carlton, K., & Ryan, M. (2004). Students' perceptions of online learning: implications for teaching. *Nurse Educator. 29*(3), 111–115.

Chambers, D. (2004). From recruitment to graduation: A whole-of-institution approach to supporting online students. *Online Journal of Distance Learning Administration, 7*(4). Retrieved September 13, 2005 from http://www.westga.edu/~distance/jmain11.html

Forman, D., Nyatanga, L., & Rich, T. (2002). E-learning and educational diversity. *Nurse Education Today, 22*(1), 76–82.

Institute for Higher Education Policy. (2000).Quality on the line: Benchmarks for success in Internet-based distance education. Retrieved August 29, 2005 from www.ihep.org/Pubs/PDF/Quality.pdf

Krueger, R. A., & Casey, M. A. (2000). *Focus groups: A practical guide for applied research* (3rd ed.). Thousand Oaks, CA: Sage Publications.

Issel, L. (2004). *Health program planning and evaluation: A practical, systematic approach for community health.* Boston: Jones & Bartlett.

Mansell, I., Bennett, G., Northway, R., Mead, D., & Moseley, L. (2004). The learning curve: The advantages and disadvantages in the use of focus groups as a method of data collection. *Nurse Researcher, 11*(4), 79–88.

McLafferty, I. (2004). Focus group interviews as a data collecting strategy. *Journal of Advanced Nursing, 48*(2), 187–194.

Mosbaek, N. L. (1999). *The lived experience of graduate nursing students in distance education.* Unpublished doctoral dissertation, The University of North Dakota, Grand Forks, ND.

Oehlkers, R. A., & Gibson, C. C. (2001). Learner support experience by RNs in a collaborative distance RN-to-BSN program. *Journal of Continuing Education in Nursing, 32*(6), 266–273.

Palloff, R. M., & Pratt, K. (1999). *Building learning communities in cyberspace: Effective strategies for the online classroom.* San Francisco: Jossey-Bass.

Thiele, J. E. (2003). Learning patterns of online students. *Journal of Nursing Education, 42*(8), 364–366.

Objectives

Upon completion of this chapter, the learner will be able to:

- Identify faculty selection factors to promote successful online program development and implementation.
- Develop a systems approach for supporting faculty engaged in offering online courses.
- Examine key elements necessary to the creation of decision rules underpinning online education.
- Identify means of reducing faculty burden through virtual student assistance.

Key Terms

Asynchronous: Descriptive of preprogrammed information that is available for transmittal or interaction at the time the user chooses and does not require real-time interaction.

Course Limits: The number of students that the instructor, in concert with academic administration, determines can be reasonably managed in a single web-based course section.

Course Section: A single group of coregistered students proceeding through organized academic content.

Decision Rules: Established tenets applied to all online course offerings.

Modular Course Offerings: Content areas divided into logical groupings and made available to online students in defined time limits (usually a period of weeks) before being closed to access.

Networking: The formation of a coordinating or support group composed of online course faculty.

Synchronous: Real-time web-based communication between instructor and student(s).

Virtual Office Hours: The posting of regular, real-time availability of an online instructor for student contact by web communication.

Workload Credit: The formal means of recognizing faculty time and effort in the development, offering, and management of an online course as other responsibilities such as course teaching, committee assignments, and clinical and research expectations are assigned.

CHAPTER SIX

Faculty Support

■ MARY ETTA MILLS

Chapter Outline

Faculty are the human capital that runs the engine of online education. These individuals are responsible for the development of innovative and timely content pertinent to students' plans of study. Student experience with online education depends on faculty being attentive to their needs and responsive to their communications. The support of faculty through careful online planning and direct involvement in creation of decision rules is critical to how faculty feel about their experience and their ability to succeed in course development, instruction, and management.

The World Wide Web offers opportunities for the delivery of nursing courses to facilitate learning on demand and learner-centered instruction. Institutions are able to establish new forms of electronic collaboration from the student to the institutional level that can facilitate major improvements in both access and learning while meeting institutional concerns about cost and quality. The development and implementation of educationally and technologically sound curricular content, while the central product of web-based distance education, is only as effective as the system's infrastructure that supports the courses and the faculty that teach them.

The selection of faculty and the development of a working group for networking and mentoring are critical to initial online program development. Efforts must be supported through support personnel with both the education and talent to assist faculty in the translation of content to an online format that uses the vast resources of the web for course enrichment. The further creation of decision rules and communication structures serves to increase efficiency and reduce faculty burden in course management.

This chapter provides a discussion of the key elements necessary for the support of faculty teaching online courses. Examples of supportive measures and processes developed and tested in practical application are presented.

SELECTION OF FACULTY

In the Beginning: Volunteers First

Diffusion of innovation literature (Rogers, 1983) supports the framework of early, middle, and late adopters of innovative technology. The diffusion of innovation involves communication of the innovation through a network of individuals and a decision on the part of one or more members to try the new measure. Based on the individual's experience with the trial, a further decision is made to adopt or reject continued use. Each individual makes a decision based on perceived characteristics of the innovation, including advantage, complexity, compatibility, trial-ability, and observability of effectiveness. Markus (1983) further proposed theories of resistance to information system implementation. He viewed resistance as a function of cognitive style or personality, issues related to the software application, and problems related to the interaction of people and systems, such as the effect on roles and responsibilities.

Organizations entering the market of online educational offerings should begin by assessing organizational readiness and resources. Individuals who are fundamental to the creation and instruction of online offerings should be consulted regarding their willingness to adopt an online education model. Furthermore, an inventory of faculty interested in participating in online education should be created. To begin, only one faculty member need be interested in putting content online, either as a hybrid course offered partially face-to-face and partially online or fully online. This person, with support, can become a champion for the entire endeavor. Success is contagious.

If a volunteer is not forthcoming, a willing participant can be developed with assistance from an internal or external consultant able to work directly with the faculty member to develop content in an online format, including PowerPoint, audiovisual, web links, and virtual experiences, to enhance student learning. There must be adequate time allowed to make this first experience a satisfying one.

Developing the course is only the first part of the process. Continuous support must be made available throughout the time that students are enrolled. Student satisfaction and a smoothly running course will be the strongest endorsements for others to participate.

In the Middle: The Jury Is Out

In *Sizing the Opportunity* (Allen & Seaman, 2003), it was noted that academic leaders at 59.6% of the institutions surveyed agreed that their faculty accepted the value of online education, leaving over 40% of institutions as neutral or in disagreement with the statement. Faculty hesitant to participate in online education may be taking a wait-and-see attitude. They are the individuals who need encouragement from support team members and from their faculty colleagues. They may also need a specific administrative decision that their course be made available online. This decision may be driven by programmatic need or by opportunities that make this accommodation desirable to the individual faculty member. Programmatic need may include requirements to increase course offering flexibility or to make an entire program of study available online. Opportunities may include increased faculty flexibility, innovative program development, external funding, or personal challenge. Often faculty who are slow adopters of online course development and instruction may also be the most talented master teachers and specialized content innovators. These individuals, having a successful first try, often receive some of the highest student evaluations.

Last but not Least: The Loyal Opposition

There are faculty who will be late adopters of innovation or, perhaps, will never move to adopt the new technology. These faculty may hold philosophic views that only face-to-face instruction adequately socializes students and provides appropriate networking opportunities. Some may feel threatened that the online course will reduce, or eliminate, their importance to the institution by moving their content into the public realm. These fears may have some legitimacy, but in reality, each course reflects the tone of its instructor, content is constantly revised, and student–faculty interaction is individualized. Expertise will also rule the day, and expert faculty well networked in the field and at the forefront of knowledge development will always be in demand.

An Embarrassment of Riches: When Everyone Wants to Participate

If the experience of online course development is a good one for faculty and meets student needs, a groundswell of demand may be created. At this point, many opportunities for placing course content online may be identified and proposed by faculty. Organizations must exercise caution to maintain adequate support for existing courses before undertaking the development of new online courses. An assessment of current course maintenance efforts must be accomplished and a determination made of additional capacity or additional resources needed. Failure to provide adequate faculty and student support for existing courses will create a system of entropy in which satisfaction decreases, the perceived workload increases, and the intent to continue participating in offering online courses decreases.

NETWORKING, FACULTY DEVELOPMENT, AND MENTORSHIP

Faculty, whether experienced or inexperienced in online education, benefit from an opportunity to compare course management and educational approaches, expand their base of knowledge, and obtain guidance from an expert focused on their progress. The report *Quality on the Line: Bechmarks for Success in Internet-based Distance Education* (Institute for Higher Education Policy, 2000) highlights several faculty support benchmarks. Among these, the most importance was placed on technical assistance to faculty in course development, assistance in the transition from classroom teaching to distance instruction, instructor training throughout the progression of the online class, and the availability of peer mentoring resources. Of these benchmarks, only technical assistance was identified as being frequently offered.

Networking begins with local support from technology designers, peers, and administrators and extends to colleagues involved in online education in other institutions and diverse professions. The formation of a coordinating group of online faculty is essential. This group should be led by someone able to plan, direct, and facilitate the progress of online course development and management and able to keep the group focused on action planning and creative resolution of course management issues and online policies relevant to concerns raised by faculty. Examples of these concerns may include faculty–student communication, management of group projects online, the number of students allowed in an online course, and faculty workload in course development and instruction.

Course Development and Management Support

The coordinating group of online faculty should begin by outlining initial plans for the development and scheduling of a program of online courses. In order to prepare faculty for their role in course development and offerings, a series of seminars may be planned. As Littman (2002) explained, teaching an online course requires a special skill set; faculty must not only know how to deliver content, but also know what content is most effective online. Faculty preparation includes the following:

● An overview of pedagogy as applied through online education.
● Orientation to teaching online courses and to supportive technology, such as the platform on which courses will be based (e.g., WebCT or Blackboard).
● The process of course development as mediated by the web.
● Case studies in course design issues.
● Faculty hands-on opportunities.

Tutorials on CD-ROMs or web-based best practices can provide faculty with a means of independent learning. Faculty development should focus on communicating online with students through bulletin boards, e-mail, and chat rooms, especially with regard to organizing discussions, providing appropriate and timely feedback, and providing clear expectations for student assignments. Faculty preparation should also include how to use basic development tools in the courseware.

Early issues to be addressed by the coordinating group may include those identified in Table 6.1.

Communication and networking among peers provides a means for sharing information, deliberating about goals and standards, and establishing plans and processes that are supportive to each individual. Interdisciplinary exchange further enhances the consideration of new perspectives and can increase access to mentoring relationships.

Some of the first support structures will also include the development of a philosophy and operational issues, such as those listed in Table 6.1.

Early Technical Concerns in Online Course Development

TABLE 6.1	ISSUES	IMPLEMENTATION
	Course access	Net account numbers for all registered students
	Course reference access	Digital library; students need a graphical web browser; identification and configuration instructions for their computers; class password for e-reserve
	Official class list	Section participants can be managed by a mass addition
	Student assistance	Help desk availability to be established
	Technology	Specific hardware and software requirements to be listed on the web for student reference
	Examination management	Decisions must be made regarding policies guiding student testing: online; site based; proctored or unproctored

Mid-Range Development Support

Once basic operations are in place, new considerations will include management of special resources necessary to enhance course quality. Fundamental course support is provided through student access to reference material. Library support to faculty for distance education initiatives is essential. Some important questions to ask the health professions reference librarian include the following:

1. Can or does your library support distance learning programs?
2. If the library currently supports distance learning, are these programs traditional courses at remote sites or web-based?
3. What types of services are available? Services may include access to an online catalog; access to digital resources such as databases, e-journals, and e-books; e-reserve; document delivery (hard copy or digital); book borrowing and shipping to remote sites; library orientations, and online courses.

Developed Programs

Regular review, evaluation, revision, and development of institutional measures to continuously improve quality are the hallmarks of developed programs. Although student evaluations of courses and faculty are critical at each level of program development, the review of aggregate evaluations that indicate the overall quality and effectiveness of a program are of equal importance. Faculty can be assisted by the automation of evaluation activities and regular analysis and feedback via systems support.

Course and faculty evaluations are essential to the development and continuous improvement of all courses. Faculty can be assisted by online tips, as illustrated in Box 6.1, that reinforce the use of a Course Evaluation Questionnaire at the completion of the semester.

Developed courses and programs may be made available to multi-institutional collectives that serve to expand opportunities to students from diverse academic and

Sample Tip 1: Using a Course Evaluation Questionnaire

Here are the steps to release your Course Evaluation Questionnaire/Faculty Evaluation Questionnaires (CEQ/FEQ) to your students taking web-based courses in Blackboard:

1. Go to the **control panel** and click **assessment manager**.
2. Click the **set availability** button next to the CEQ/FEQ survey.
3. Under option 1, click **yes**.
4. When the screen refreshes, note the default selections and then click **submit**.

Suggestion: Modify the announcement and make it either **permanent** or **displayed until the end of the semester**. Also, please note that the CEQ/FEQ records answers anonymously (names are not associated with surveys; however, the online gradebook will reflect that the CEQ/FEQ has been taken and submitted by a student).

geographic environments. For example, the Southern Regional Education Board Electronic Campus (http://www.electroniccampus.org/) makes courses available to students from a wide range of universities. Students may enroll in online courses offered by colleges as part of this collaborative effort, pay the offering institution's tuition, and have the course recorded on their home school's transcript. The availability of courses makes it possible for a college to build a student's program of study without assuming responsibility for the time, effort, and cost that it might require to develop and offer a course for which there would be limited enrollment.

COMMUNICATION TO FACULTY

Direct and frequent communication to faculty is an important means of providing ongoing support. Regular tips such as the following provide faculty with unsolicited assistance and validate that they are not the only individuals with a need for specific information. The sample tip presented in Box 6.2 is an example of a communication from the instructional design technologist to online faculty offered as a helpful hint in anticipation of their need, and a reminder to check student engagement in the course, at the beginning of the semester.

The management of the electronic gradebook shown in Box 6.3 is another Sample Tip providing direct assistance to faculty.

PERSONNEL SUPPORT

Technical and program management support is critical to providing faculty with the expertise necessary to design, implement, and manage the educational and administrative development and maintenance of online courses. Essential to the process are an instructional design technologist and an online program manager. These individuals provide direct assistance to faculty developing and teaching online courses.

Sample Tip 2: Example of a Communication From the Instructional Design Technologist

BOX 6.2

FYI: Are you wondering if your students have logged on successfully? Here's how you can tell:

1. Click **control panel**.
2. Under the **assessment** area, click **course statistics**.
3. Scroll down to section 3 and make sure **Yes** is selected.
4. Scroll down and click **submit**.

Then you'll see a detailed analysis of what they've been doing. If they haven't posted to the Introductions discussion board yet, encourage them to do so by posting an announcement.

Sample Tip 3: Management of Electronic Gradebooks

FYI: It is strongly recommended that Blackboard electronic gradebooks be either **printed** (or **exported**) whenever **new grades are posted**. Once inside your Blackboard course, here are the steps for each method:

Printing gradebooks:

1. Click **control panel** and then click **electronic gradebook**.
2. Click **spreadsheet view**.
3. From the Internet Explorer menu bar, click **File** and then select **Print**.
4. Save hard copy in a secure place.

Exporting gradebook and importing into an Excel spreadsheet:

1. Click **control panel** and then click **electronic gradebook**.
2. Click **export gradebook**.
3. Right-click on **save exported gradebook** and select **save target as.**
4. Save electronic copy in a secure place.

(Note: After saving the file, open **Microsoft Excel**, click **File** menu and select **Open**.)

Instructional Design Technologist

The development of course content into an online format requires reconceptualization of information delivery and innovative use of technology to expand the possibilities offered by web resources. The role of the instructional design technologist is to:

● Work with faculty to organize course content into a format for online delivery in consideration of good learning principles.
● Develop clear definition within course modules through consistent syllabi and content delivery.
● Provide structure to audiovisual material such as PowerPoint slides and video streaming through consideration of clarity, presentation quality, and efficiency of information portrayal.
● Assist in the identification of web site links related to specific areas of course content.
● Develop adjunctive media in support of the course content in collaboration with the faculty.
● Develop course-related student support infrastructure such as exam schedule posting, student enrollment list, and course tracking.
● Serve as consultant and mentor to help faculty incorporate creative structured and unstructured learning opportunities.

Online Program Manager

To coordinate the administrative systems and ensure quality of online programs, an online program manager is essential. Responsibilities of the online program manager include identifying issues, developing strategies, and working with online course faculty to make recommendations for the development and support of the program. Some of the basic duties of the online program manager are to:

- Produce written reports and make administrative presentations.
- Chair meetings on issues and problems related to the online program.
- Seek and evaluate information from various sources and make recommendations for developing support systems for students and faculty.
- Plan and implement professional development programs for faculty to convert courses from face-to-face to online format.
- Collaborate with faculty to resolve technical issues.

As the number of online courses increases and the level of sophistication of material used to deliver the course becomes more complex, additional personnel will be necessary to support the effort.

Technical support should be available on a round-the-clock basis with an institutional or contractual arrangement for troubleshooting and problem-solving recommendations. Students may be asked to try to resolve problems themselves, by using online help menus, manuals, and web resources, before contacting faculty or the help desk.

CREATING DECISION RULES

Decision rules establish the premise on which the operating policies and procedures relevant to online course construction and management are based. These rules are the guiding principles for what is—and what is not—allowed and expected in the establishment, implementation, and expected outcomes of online courses. Within this context, decision rules must address issues of student examinations, faculty–student communication, course completion expectations, and course registration volume capacity.

Student Examinations

Divisive situations between faculty may be avoided through a clear determination of standard mechanisms to be used to evaluate student performance. Although it may be desirable to establish one means of testing, not all course content realistically lends itself to the same method of evaluation. Less important than establishing one standard method of testing is the clarification of methods and processes that will be considered part of the compendium of techniques. Table 6.2 presents some examples of methods for consideration that are further discussed in Chapter Ten.

Frequency of Communication With Students

Student inquiries to the course instructor outside of virtual office hours may involve questions, comments, or advice that the student considers important in the short-term. Online course policy should include the frequency to which these communications should be responded and should be so noted in the online policies available to students. Ideally, responses to students should be made within 24 to 48 hours of the inquiry. This exemplar

Examination Methods

METHOD	CONSIDERATIONS	APPROACHES
Unproctored online exam	Academic integrity and test security	Develop large test item pool and randomize test question selection. Print lock exams so they cannot be printed. Automate time limit on exam. Have student sign honor contract. Administer narrative exam.
Proctored online exam	Faculty test management time	Set standard guidelines for identifying and obtaining a proctor. Devise a standard form for proctors and the student testing contract. Provide specific information and instructions regarding exams in the course syllabus. Give students options regarding taking proctored exams at a center or arranging an individual proctor. Offer exam scheduling options. Recruit student proctors.
On-site examinations	Location access and support	Obtain distant sites for proctoring. Contract service. Preschedule examinations.

requires that faculty be online and posting messages 5 out of 7 days a week and providing regular feedback to students. Assignments should be graded within 1 week. To achieve this, faculty must have broadband or high-speed Internet connections and must be able to access the school system from a distance.

Virtual Office Hours

Regular availability of an instructor to communicate with online students in real time must be established at the beginning of the course. Many instructors establish a 2-hour block of time each week when they will be online for direct synchronous student interaction. This opportunity for direct one-to-one exchange is essential so that students can seek clarification, additional information, or advice relative to the course content or academic progression.

Modular Offerings

A decision may be made to offer course content in an open time frame format in which the student can complete the entire course at any time. Courses may also be structured as modules intended to be completed within specific time frames. These modular offerings carry defined objectives and are available to students during a specified part of the semester. The rationale for a modular approach is to ensure that students keep up with coursework and fully participate and interact with other students in the course. Because web sites often change their content, a modular approach is advantageous in ensuring that articles or online newsletters will be available to students. A modular approach requires that modules be posted on time and that the assignment of due dates be clearly stated. PowerPoint slides and syllabi must have the same title as the modules.

Course Registration Limits

Although the number of students enrolled in a course may certainly vary, the upper limit is recommended at 20 to 25. Course limits should be decided jointly by colleagues teaching online courses, registrars, and academic administrators. If the course cap limit is reached, students should be added only by the instructor teaching the course. The lower limit of enrollment in an online course should be determined by resource allocation needs and recapturing of expense; generally, enrollment must be eight or higher to make the course feasible. The cost of funding and effort of an instructor for a smaller number of students may not be reasonable in view of the need to cover other larger online or face-to-face course sections.

FACULTY WORKLOAD CREDIT

Development and management of an online course consumes faculty time and effort. Faculty frequently express that more time is necessary for online courses than for face-to-face courses. The work is seemingly transparent because of the behind-the-scenes preparation of PowerPoint, video streaming, audiovisual, web linkage identification, case studies, interactive scenarios, and re-envisioning of content delivery. Once the course is online and students are registered, time is required for review of student participation, faculty–student communication, virtual office hours, and grading of coursework. The larger the number of students enrolled in the course, the more time is required of faculty.

Consideration should be given to recognizing faculty time requirements for course development, instruction for each online course, and size of class. Course development takes the same amount of effort as actually offering the course. The size of the class must be determined based on the nature of the course, the level of communication, follow-up, evaluation required per student, and the experience and preparation of the instructor.

PREEMPTING STUDENT QUESTIONS

An important method of supporting faculty is reducing the number of student inquiries that they must manage by providing proactive, web-based asynchronous information.

Orientation

Student orientation to online courses is essential to enumerate the competencies, skills, and resources students will need to actively participate in online learning. This orientation should be delivered online to all students who enroll in an online learning activity. The orientation should be a series of modules, exercises, and required reading that can be divided into topics. Content may include: computer hardware and software; basic computer skills; platform navigation; online learning, including a self-assessment quiz; Internet etiquette; identification of available online resources, such as purchasing books and course material; a virtual writing center; a virtual counseling center; academic advising; issues of confidentiality; a virtual library; and the use of help sites and problem solving. The availability of course previews will further assist in circumventing questions regarding the nature, objectives, and requirements of the course.

Registration

Before being registered for an online course, students should be oriented to online education processes and expectations. User identification and passwords should have been issued, HELP resources and contact information made available, and exam schedules and proctoring policy communicated.

In the first 2 weeks of the semester, course rosters should be run every other day and compared to the online course enrollments. This will enable the course administrator to contact students who may not actively search out information regarding log-in instructions in a timely fashion. Because course rosters can vary dramatically in the beginning weeks, it is suggested that any group projects be delayed until the fourth week, when groups can be created without major shuffling.

Exams

If exams for a course are proctored, times and locations of the exams should be scheduled before the semester begins. Students should be given notification of these times in the course syllabus. For those students who do not reside in the state from which the course emanates, policies for obtaining a proctor should be available online. The Virginia Tech web site offers a resource for proctor procedures (http://www.iddl.vt.edu/handbook/proctor.php).

To the extent that proctors can be organized and students given exam appointments or offered online exam options, faculty can be relieved of having to arrange and personally monitor students' test taking. As part of reducing faculty burden during the course, due dates for any course requirements should also be scheduled before the course begins and communicated within the online course syllabus.

More labor intensive but less subject to academic misconduct is the assignment of narrative papers on assigned topics. This can work especially well for graduate students and for courses that might be dually listed as undergraduate and graduate offerings. In the latter event, graduate students are usually assigned an additional paper beyond that expected of undergraduates, which has more complex expectations, such as a critical analysis of the literature and applications to nursing and health care. Although papers do not require a proctor, they do require an assessment by faculty that the work is that of the student and does not involve plagiarism. This can be accomplished by conducting a search of key terms or phrases in Google.

CONCLUSION

The best online course development and infrastructure will not substitute for creative, responsive, and knowledgeable faculty supported by clear decision rules for course management. Faculty are not inherently prepared to teach in an online format. Support for faculty development in online education techniques and methods and ongoing mentorship are essential to the preparation and growth of faculty expertise in this teaching domain. Recognition of the workload involved in creating, instructing, and managing an online course is essential. Likewise, the identification of a reasonable cap for student enrollment in online courses must be determined based on course requirements and content difficulty requiring more instructor effort.

Students planning to participate in online education require preparation prior to beginning coursework. Orientation to the structure of course participation, including navigation of courseware, expectations for participation, technical problem solving, and management of course requirements, is critical. A combination of well-prepared faculty and students will promote a satisfying learning environment.

■ LEARNING ACTIVITIES

● Initiate a web search to identify online education programs that offer a virtual orientation, course previews, and student self-assessment tools.
● Conduct an e-reference literature search on e-learning faculty support.
● Identify and interview an instructional design technologist regarding roles and responsibilities and the most effective means of working collaboratively in offering a web-based course.
● Critically review online strategies (debates, discussion groups, exams, assignments) for student evaluation.

REFERENCES

Allen, I. E., & Seaman, J. (2003). *Sizing the opportunity: The quality and extent of online education in the United States, 2002 and 2003* (Vol. 2). Needham, MA: Sloan Center for Online Education.

Institute for Higher Education Policy. (2000). *Quality on the line: Benchmarks for success in Internet-based distance education.* Washington, D.C.: Institute for Higher Education Policy.

Littman, M. (2002). Teaching the teacher. *University Business*, Sept. 2002, 49–53.

Rogers, E. (1983). *Diffusion of innovation* (3rd ed.). New York: Free Press.

Markus, M. (1983). Power, politics, and MIS implementation. *Communication of the ACM, 26*(6), 430–444.

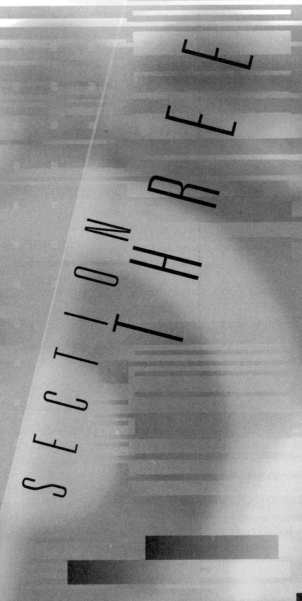

SECTION THREE

**Curricular
Considerations**

Objectives

Upon completion of this chapter, the learner will be able to:

- Select a pedagogic model for the further development of online educational programs.
- Critically evaluate models of online education in consideration of academic program philosophy and organizational requirements, resources, or limitations.
- Plan online health education course delivery consistent with outcome and regulatory requirements of health care providers.
- Design a curriculum in consideration of achievement of learning outcomes.

Key Terms

Competency Testing: Formal evaluation of learned skills and skill application.

Critical Thinking: Purposeful, self-regulatory judgment that results in interpretation, analysis, evaluation, and inference, as well as explanation of the evidential, conceptual, methodological, criteriological, or contextual considerations on which that judgment is based (Facione, 1990, p. 3).

Pedagogy: The art of teaching; principles of education used in constructing methods to facilitate learning.

Standardized Learning Outcomes: Uniform expectations for knowledge acquisition at the conclusion of a course or program of study.

Time-Designed: Course instruction planned to meet specific calendar requirements.

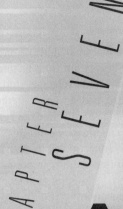

CHAPTER SEVEN

Academic Programs

■ MARY ETTA MILLS AND
DOROTHEA McDOWELL

Chapter Outline

cademic programs are designed to expand the knowledge base of students through a variety of learning experiences. Although passive learning may result from lectured material, active learning involves interactivity through communication exchange, student use of multiple information sources, exercises, skill development, and activities. In the interest of developing collegial networks, proficiency in knowledge application, and critical thinking ability, online education for health care professionals must be carefully constructed and delivered. Because much of health professions education is, by its nature, intended to build on previous knowledge and experience, it is especially important to consider the relationship of models of pedagogy, instructional strategies, and technology, in the context of educational outcomes in health science education.

PEDAGOGICAL MODELS FROM INSTRUCTIVISM TO CONSTRUCTIVISM AND BEYOND

Theory, whether liked or not, is necessary to view work in online education from a broader perspective. Theory helps build on the known while seeing new worlds and can assist in effective use of time in development and delivery of online materials. Several models to link learning theories to online education are currently being proposed (Anderson, 2004; Dabbagh, 2004; Shea, Pickett, & Pelz, 2003). A review of the more prevalent learning and related theories will assist with understanding applications in online education.

Instructivism uses the approach of passive learning and relies heavily on instructor dominated didactic teaching with traditional examinations based on delivered content. Factual information may be best taught using an instructivistic approach. In under-graduate nursing education, didactic information on a topic such as health promotion in children may best be taught using this approach. The childhood immunization schedule, for example, is factual information that is easily taught using an instructivist approach. In an online education environment, this model could use streaming video, audio, textual, or mixed media of information delivery. Supplementary materials might include a note taking guide, self-testing quizzes with immediate feedback for remediation, and prescribed text and reference materials.

Constructivism assumes that each learner has developed an individual understanding of subjects and ideas influenced by their perspective, personality, and background. This model assumes that an individual will relate new information to the background knowledge already attained through other life experiences. A sense of an online community that promotes interaction among students and educators has been identified as helpful in obtaining educational outcomes in the constructivist view (Conrad, 2002). The constructivist approach is supportive of student-centered learning and is especially appropriate for students who are already licensed professionals such as registered nurses in a baccalaureate completion program, graduate students, or participants in continuing professional education programs. By building on pre-existing knowledge and experiences, learners integrate new knowledge to develop new constructs. Online education may follow a constructivist approach through: problem-based learning; synchronous and asynchronous communication between students and between student and instructor; discovery methods by which students search, locate, and evaluate reference resources; and individualized mentored projects. Instructor-guided discussions based on case scenarios to apply concepts of community health nursing is an example of the application of constructivism in nursing education.

Transactional Distance is a theory of the pedagogy of distance education (Moore & Kearsley, 2005), of which online learning is a part. "Transactional Distance is the gap of understanding and communication between the teachers and learners caused by geographic distance that must be bridged through distinctive procedures in instructional design and the facilitation of interaction" (Moore & Kearsley, p. 223). Interestingly, this distance can be seen in any educational event, even in face-to-face situations. Although not a traditional learning theory, transactional distance theory has been widely discussed and applied to online education.

The theory of transactional distance includes two clusters of teaching behaviors: dialogue and structure. The idea of dialogue is based on constructivism theories of learning in which a dialogue between the teacher and student results in a shift of control of the learning process to the student (Moore & Kearsley, 2005). Structure is the term used to delineate elements in the course's design such as case studies, exercises, and content units. The structure of an online course is determined by the following: the teacher's educational philosophy; the level of the student, such as undergraduate versus graduate; nature of the content; and the available communication techniques.

In conclusion, models are being created as a result of technologic capabilities that allow online education to maximize a variety of learning theories and instructional methods. Technology-based interactivity has unique capabilities such as video streaming, online reference libraries, web-based doors to agencies and experiences with 24-hour, 7 days-a-week access, chat rooms and web logs (blogs) to network with other students, faculty and global experts. Using these portals (both faculty directed and student discovered) allows an enhanced learning environment that maximizes student-centered learning. The integration of a wide variety of learning resources that is both faculty and student initiated can create a unique experience for each student. One of these models will be explored next.

Online Learning Model for Curriculum Development

In order to link theory to practice, a model that identifies the basic components of online learning and the direction of interaction between the components is helpful. In the area of online education, several models have been posited. One simple three-component model (Figure 7.1) that emphasizes the recursive and transformative interaction between pedagogical models, learning technologies, and instructional strategies has been presented by Dabbagh (2004, p. 42). This author presents these three components as equals so that any one component will not be seen as more important than another. Dabbagh (2004) also states that the bidirectional arrows give the online course designer flexibility to begin from any point in the model and then proceed in either direction.

A novice online course designer might begin constructing a course by first familiarizing himself or herself with the available course management system. Once the capabilities

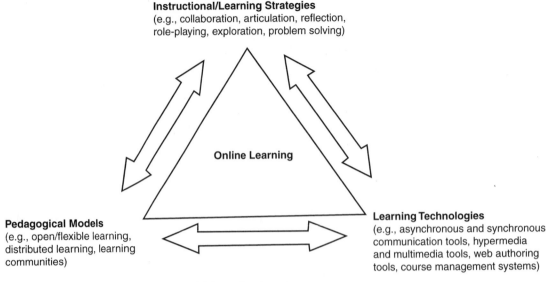

Instructional/Learning Strategies
(e.g., collaboration, articulation, reflection,
role-playing, exploration, problem solving)

Online Learning

Pedagogical Models
(e.g., open/flexible learning,
distributed learning, learning
communities)

Learning Technologies
(e.g., asynchronous and synchronous
communication tools, hypermedia
and multimedia tools, web authoring
tools, course management systems)

FIGURE 7.1 A three-component model for online learning.

of the system are known, learning strategies are identified concurrently with the identification of appropriate pedagogical models. Another course designer may want to start with instructional strategies that have been successful in the past and then progress to identifying what learning technologies are appropriate for these instructional strategies. The course designer could then tie the course together by identifying the pedagogical model that is being used.

This model is of particular interest because of its flexibility in application and its simplicity. As each of the three components evolves, the model will not become outdated. The area of learning technologies particularly is evolving so rapidly, it is difficult to keep pace. This model affords the new technologies a place to be included. The same is true of instructional or learning strategies. This area is explored next.

INSTRUCTIONAL STRATEGIES: USE OF COMMUNICATION VENUES

Distance education, including online learning, depends on well thought-out communication venues. Asynchronous communication in which time of interaction is flexible and accessible to students depends on use of a rich array of mechanisms that support learning. Given that students have different learning preferences, such as visual, auditory, and kinesthetic, the use of varied means of communication becomes essential.

Visual learners acquire an advantage when content is delivered through venues such as text, graphics, and video. Auditory learners tend to respond to sound and voice communication. Kinesthetic learners favor approaches that use motor skills and hands-on activities.

Online instruction that integrates these approaches has the effect of mediating differences in learning style and can assist in the ability to optimally interact with, and retain, content knowledge. This concept is consistent with that of universal design whereby courses are planned to be accessible to students and instructors with a wide range of abilities and disabilities. Universal design is defined by the Center for Universal Design at North Carolina State University as "the design of products and environments to be usable by all people, to the greatest extent possible, with the need for adaptation or specialized design" (http://www.design.ncsu.edu/cud/univ_design/ud.htm). One of the key principles of this design is that it accommodates a wide range of individual preferences and abilities (Anders & Fechtner, 1992).

Visual Communication

The first online challenge often involves capturing images, video, class lectures, and other types of content for access over the web. This may also include text-based resources such as discussion boards, chat rooms, bulletin boards, e-mail, graphics, databases, animations, and simulations to promote active learning. Multimedia files have a combination of visual and audio presentations. In designing visual components it is essential that some basic standards are considered, including the following:

- Organization and readability of text-based documents, including clarity of content as well as of visualization through font size, spacing, and screen density (the amount of information on any one screen).
- Data tables with clear column and row headers; frame titles to help the user understand the frame's purpose.
- Clear navigation links.
- Verification of validity of hyperlinks and availability of archives.
- User control over the timing of content changes.
- Match syllabus and module titles.

These standards will be useful in addressing some frequently identified student-related difficulties such as reading PowerPoint slides and attachments, accessing web-based resources identified in the course modules, and logical progression and integration of content.

Development of visual communication requires one or more multimedia stations that are equipped with speakers, a headset, video card, and RealMedia authoring and development package. This allows for both broadcasting and digitizing live presentations, and digitizing authorized educational videos (when copyright has been released). A mini video recorder is useful so that the video camera does not have to be attached to the multimedia station while digitizing video. In his article "Virtually Perfect," Joseph Panettieri (2004) discusses the list of requirements to build a video presentation system that involves cameras, video capture cards, network pipelines, servers, digital displays, projection systems, and whiteboards. The level of equipment required will depend on the extent of online production anticipated.

Auditory Communication

Although auditory communication is generally produced in conjunction with a visual component, it is possible to produce some modules or portions of modules that are entirely auditory. This may take the form of content review with a verbal review and description of content in a lecture style and may be accompanied by aids such as a note taking guide or other content outline. For skill development, web sites that offer heart sounds and breath sounds may be produced with verbal introductions and descriptions that precede and summarize the actual auditory symptoms of the physical examination.

Kinesthetic Communication

Motor skills and hands on activities that are application oriented are a means of allowing the learner to practice knowledge gained through other communication modalities. Online programs and interactive software are able to facilitate the development of critical thinking and application skills through simulated client cases, virtual physical assessment, and practice-based education and resource referencing.

An example of skill building using practical application is *Virtual Stethoscope*, developed at McGill University. This program includes practice in identifying normal and abnormal cardiac and respiratory conditions through sound, text, and visual representation. Learners have an opportunity to gain experience in identifying heart and breath sounds through auscultation using a virtual stethoscope and to conduct a physical examination on a virtual patient.

Virtual practice further permits students and professionals to development and fine tune skills that might not otherwise be available. One case in point is a virtual mass spectrometry lab offered on the web site developed by Carnegie Mellon University and the University of Pittsburgh (Carnevale, 2003). The program gives students an opportunity to experience how the equipment works by practicing with four online case studies. The equipment can be adjusted to focus on different molecular tests.

Using a combination of online learning and on-site practice application or return demonstration offers another means of motor skill development. An online physical assessment course, for example, may present all content online while requiring that students arrange to be videotaped in a randomly selected application. The videotape is subsequently mailed to the instructor who completes the review and evaluation for purposes of grading and feedback.

BALANCING AND OPTIMIZING LEARNING STRATEGIES

The most complex design of online learning involves balancing the various communication venues. The process outlined in Box 7.1 demonstrates the combination of text-based, audiovisual, and kinesthetic learning approaches.

Text-Based and Audiovisual Presentations (Faculty-Directed)

Online course presentation first incorporates material that is directed to the student from the instructor as introductory information. The course syllabus is presented in a printable form with well-defined content modules and completion timelines. If modules will be

Balancing Web-Based Learning Approaches

BOX 7.1

Text-Based and Audiovisual Presentations (Faculty-Directed)

● Course syllabus includes content topic by module and time lines.
● Define course requirements including deliverables, type, and frequency of student interaction, and expected faculty response.
● Identify content resources, including e-texts, e-references, virtual experiences, cases, and such.

Synchronous Text and Audio Access

● Virtual office hours via e-mail or voice.

Text-Based and Audiovisual Presentations (Student Interaction)

● PowerPoint and video presentations of content with audio overlay or concurrent.
● Hyperlinks to virtual field visits, agencies, and resources.
● Case-based logic tree scenarios of virtual practice decisions and actions.

Written Assignments

● Student assignment of case analysis and problem-based learning exercises.
● Papers and critiques.
● Simulation-based data analysis.

Kinesthetic Experiences

● Virtual practice of motor skills such as physical assessment for application.
● Competency testing using virtual physical exams.

time-limited in availability, this information must be made explicit. Text-based information may be accompanied by an introductory video that provides a preview of the course content by the instructor and expectations for course completion. Although each module will incorporate its own reference resources, electronic references for use across the entire course and preparatory work such as familiarization with reference agencies and documents should be included in the text-based syllabus and referred to during the overview. Each online course should provide easy access to a help desk in the event of technology problems requiring assistance by the student. Even with experience, students may encounter difficulty with the use of an electronic drop box for the return of assignments, effective linkage to external resources, and use of simulations. Ancillary means of communication should also be defined such as telephone contact numbers, and times of real and virtual office hours. The level of interaction between students, and between faculty and students should also be made clear. Chat rooms are text-based and should be monitored and responded to by the instructor. Bulletin boards of notices and related class communication are also text-based and must be maintained in a current state. Occasionally, small groups may have visual contact among members and faculty through the use of web cameras on their home computers. If this is desirable for seminars, the expectation must be included in the course description and syllabus as it represents an additional student purchase requirement.

Synchronous Text and Audio Access

Virtual office hours via e-mail and voice will occur in real time and is important for direct communication that best benefits from direct dialogue and problem solving without a time lapse. Because online courses offer flexibility in how students time the completion of course requirements, there continues to be a need for predictable direct access to the instructor.

Text-Based and Audiovisual Presentations (Student Interaction)

Course content is optimally presented using a variety of blended presentation methods including text-based and audiovisual for student interaction. This may include the more traditional PowerPoint and video presentation with accompanying sound. The combination of a recorded voice with digital photos, video clips and slides, or streaming audio-video brings the presentation to life. Faculty may make CDs available for students to purchase that include video clips and/or other audiovisual enhancements. This is particularly useful if students are accessing the course via a dial-up modem. Multimedia allows the student to visit remote sites through a virtual tour of field settings and agencies, and hyperlinks provide additional resources beyond the traditional walls of the classroom. For example, government web sites such as www.nih.gov or www. medicare.gov provide invaluable primary information regarding active clinical trials research, disease process references, health care payment systems, and medical and hospital coverage issues.

Case-based logic tree scenarios of virtual practice problems requiring decisions and actions are especially valuable to student learning in that they require a demonstration of knowledge acquisition and can be used to develop enhanced competencies or to evaluate current actions based in critical thinking. For example, cases may be built around issues such as emergency administration of epinephrine, respiratory assessment, and emergency room triage. These cases are developed around a primary health care scenario in which a provider must assess, plan, take action to intervene, and evaluate. The approach requires a blended model of video, access to text-based data such as lab values, and the possibility of student-created projections of data to simulate expected effect of actions. The multitrack program fully explains each of several principle decisions that can be made and acted on by the student. In a triage situation, for example, the student may be presented with the emergency room setting and introduced to staff and several patients identifying themselves as needing emergency care. The student is expected to select the patient needing immediate intervention after hearing and seeing each patient's presenting symptoms. The student can select from among several possible interventions and the program responds with the effect of that decision and offers an opportunity to explore the selected patient or another patient further. As a recursive program, the student receives immediate feedback on his decisions and is referred to additional resource information for review or reference.

The blending of communication venues with automatic feedback makes it possible for active learning to take place. Use of interactive audiovisual and text-based communication can assist students to acquire a better understanding of content regardless of their learning styles and more closely approximates their interaction with a real event.

Written Assignments

The creation of written assignments requires students to synthesize content and to logically develop an idea reflective of, or further exploring, content and issues raised in the course. Online courses can draw on case analysis and problem-based cases as well as exercises requiring in-depth conceptualization, exploration, and evaluation of content. Web logs are one constructivist avenue to explore to assist students in case analysis (Maag, 2005). In order for students to have adequate time to synthesize the content, many courses indicate that students should expect to spend at least 6 hours a week working on course content and requirements. Certainly face-to-face courses also use these techniques; however, integrated access to wide-ranging resources and multimedia support to demonstrate the cases offer a unique opportunity to online students.

Interactive, data-based simulations permit students to create and test potential actions or research results and to determine optimal actions that are quantitatively supportable. Examples of this type of data might include ambulatory census numbers by specialty and by day, the projection of staffing levels to provide adequate care, and the financial impact that might result given salary expenditures and patient care revenues. Data analysis and the written report will demand application of many concepts and critical thought processes using a range of content, from research to management and clinical decision making.

Kinesthetic Experiences

Embedded within specific courses are opportunities for the development of practice skills. Courses such as physical assessment, biology, and chemistry can include virtual lab sessions in conjunction with text-based and audiovisual communication. The opportunity to build lab sessions directly into the content area in which they are most able to demonstrate the principles under review is an immediate advantage for students in that they can integrate application and content immediately and revisit the application at any time. Simulated experiences on the web can include everything from the dissection of a frog to the assessment of cranial nerves through optical examination.

Building online course modules takes innovative conceptualization of what the learner outcomes and competencies must be and an exploration of what is already available through accessible hyperlinks and what must be developed. Careful construction of opportunities to develop and use motor skills is particularly demanding and requires specialized design and production assistance due to the demand for interactivity that can result in accessing and potentially moving or changing web-based objects during the exercise.

As competency testing increasingly becomes an expectation, standardized tests are incorporating these methods. One example is the Registered Nurse Licensure Examination offered by the National Council of State Board. This test is now incorporating questions that require students to move a cursor to the appropriate site of an anatomical projection in response to questions regarding physical assessment.

SPECIFIC CONSIDERATIONS FOR ONLINE HEALTH SCIENCES EDUCATION

There are several factors to consider in selecting courses for an online format. The factors shown in Box 7.2 can be useful in determining courses to receive priority for development.

A needs assessment should be conducted to determine the market demand, especially the level of growth that could be anticipated if a course or program were placed online. Consideration must be given to the number of students who might shift to online resulting in no net increase in enrollment. Although this would not necessarily be a detractor, the result may have implications for the number of face-to-face course sections to be offered or the relative frequency of course or program offerings over an academic year.

The development of an online course or program will require resources not only for start-up, but also for long-term sustainability. An assessment must be made of faculty availability and the level of their expertise to instruct and guide learners in an online format. The availability of staff to support placement of courses into an online format must also be considered. An instructional designer will be critical to this process. This individual not only will facilitate faculty in developing and producing the online offering, but also will be an integral member of the instructional team necessary to assist in technical problem solving, as well as fostering a responsive student environment for online learning. This may take the form of responding to student questions or requests specific to the technical requirements of interfacing with course material and ensuring a high quality online course structure. Monitoring of process and problems will be important to continuous quality improvement. This level of support has budgetary implications that must be projected and a funding plan developed or external funding identified. Development and maintenance of high quality online instruction does come with additional expenses. See Chapter Two for a thorough discussion of this topic.

Course Selection Factors for Online Development

BOX 7.2

- Relation of the course or program to strategic initiatives of the school.
- Results of needs assessment regarding potential market and enrollment projection.
- Resources required to initiate and sustain the course online.
- Ability of online format to support course requirements.
- Fit of the online course into the overall program of study.
- Expense for students in addition to cost per credit.
- Ability to meet requirements of accrediting and certifying bodies when delivering courses or a program of study.
- Compliance with quality indicators established by professional groups.
- Number of courses that would be needed online to support the curriculum.
- Which existing online courses would be part of the curriculum or plan of study.

The design of student learning evaluation needs to be carefully considered. Objective testing of content needs to be secure. This can be managed through preceptored testing in an arrangement made by the student and formally contracted through the faculty with the preceptor or through an identified testing center. The evaluation of active learning will more often involve written case reports and analysis of problems or scenarios that are graded by the instructor.

The fit of an online course into the overall curriculum program of study will determine the extent to which students will be able to add flexibility to their plan of study or to complete all academic degree requirements through online learning. Development of a single, freestanding course may help to reduce scheduling problems for students and meet a need for flexibility. However, this single course approach should be used judiciously in that it is additive to the schedule of course offerings but may not assist in increasing overall student enrollment. Alternatively, developing online capacity in consideration of a complete curricula program plan will produce a different strategic plan that opens the possibility of increasing the reach of the program to rural and other distant sites. Another possibility would be the creation of an interinstitutional collaboration by which courses would be developed and shared for student access to support otherwise divergent plans of study.

Accrediting and certifying bodies expect to be notified of the availability of online programs and assured that the quality of education and ability to meet academic objectives for health professions education and outcome competencies will be equivalent to those approved in the on-site, face-to-face instructional format. This expectation includes meeting the competencies of professional groups established for specific specialties the school may identify for purposes of accreditation or certification review.

It should be noted that regional accreditation is important in that some institutions do not accept credit transfer of courses from nationally accredited institutions, which are usually for-profit colleges and universities (Carnevale, 2002). Individual institutions can decide which transfer credits to accept. Some distance education programs, such as the University of Phoenix and the University of Maryland University College, do not have this problem because they have regional accreditation. The issue centers on the expectation that transfer course credits must meet standards that are equivalent to those offered by the accepting institution.

Clinical and Lab Content and Management

One of the most interesting and practical applications of the Internet is the capability of providing users with learning opportunities involving interactive exercises and virtual experience. The web has become a tool for self-directed learning that allows expansion and enhancement of clinical skills. The advantage of this media is the ability to explore information of practical use and to gain experience where and when it is convenient to the user and as often as necessary until the skill is mastered.

An example of web-based sites for skill building can be found by using the Google Web Directory and searching on health > nursing > specialties. Some of the specialties included are community health, critical care, emergency, geriatrics, midwifery, neonatal, neuroscience, obstetrics, gynecology, pediatrics, and wound care. Some of the sites supply actual practice and skill building opportunities with presentations varying from narratives to interactive multimedia programs. Many are provided at no charge, while others involve a registration fee.

The importance of assessing the quality of the program being accessed cannot be overemphasized. Misinformation can lead to serious errors. The capacity of the Internet for wide distribution of information makes accuracy critical. It is essential that users take the time to evaluate web-based programs before depending on them for skill building.

The determination as to whether course requirements can be met in an online format must be considered. For example, what will be the implications for clinical requirements? In some cases, such as health assessment, it may be possible to conduct the entire course in an online format by using virtual assessment learning scenarios that are available on the web in conjunction with audio and video streaming or available on a CD that is packaged with the textbook. Students may provide return demonstrations by being videotaped in an appropriate environment and returning the tapes to the instructor for review and evaluation.

As online clinical curricula are designed, strategies that promote critical thinking in learners need to be included. Research identifying specific strategies that contribute to critical thinking skills and dispositions is lacking. In an effort to promote critical thinking in online education, the results, or lack of results, in research findings suggest a rationale for designing curricula around problem-based learning that demands reflection of understanding or questioning of information rather than reiterative memorization. Applied to online instructional strategies, this would suggest use of case analysis, questions requiring the identification and use of multiple resources, simulation, and analysis.

Courses that involve hands-on clinical such as community health will still need a preceptored clinical environment, but students would be able to complete content through the online format. The preceptorship would be arranged in the student's local geographic area and the logistics of managing this arrangement, including supervision and evaluation, would need to be considered before promising total availability to students, regardless of their location. The preceptored experience would also give students an opportunity to learn and practice verbal presentation skills that would be more difficult in the typical online format.

INCORPORATING ONLINE AND TRADITIONAL COURSES INTO A COMMON CURRICULUM

The blending of online and traditional face-to-face courses within the curriculum can offer students scheduling flexibility that would otherwise not be available. The key is to make a strategic and operational plan regarding the best way to accomplish academic objectives.

Some considerations for selecting courses to be placed online are shown in Box 7.3. A strategic decision must be made as to the overall academic program goal regarding the use of online courses. Will an entire program be made available online? Will selected courses be offered in an online format, and will these same courses also be offered face-to-face? Will there be restrictions on who can register for online courses? For courses offered in two formats, online and face-to-face, how will course expectations be made equivalent?

Whether the decision is to offer selected courses only in an online format or to create added access by developing courses online while maintaining face-to-face sections as

Selection Criteria for Incorporating Online Courses Into a Common Curriculum

- Registration projection
- Faculty interest and expertise
- Content level difficulty and level of student
- Course sequence
- Course requirements
- Valuation requirement for personal interaction

well, one of the first selection decisions is to establish what courses have the most potential for sustainable registration. For example, if a course is required in both an RN to BSN program and a traditional BSN program, the number of students available to take the online offering will be greater than that of a course only required for a subset of students. The development of courses that maximize the potential registration also will have the best return on investment.

In order to ensure equivalency between online and traditional courses, development and offering of the course by a faculty member interested in online education who also instructs the face-to-face version will help to give the project the stimulus it needs for creativity and consistent expectations across sections. It is useful to begin online course development with a beginning level course for an identified program. This will give students the possibility of gaining experience with online courses early in their program of study and will enhance their interactivity and success with future online courses.

Course sequencing evaluation will assist in constructing a plan by which courses can be selected for development into an online format. In this case, it is important to consider the requirement for any prerequisite or corequisite courses, course flow, and courses that create a related track of information such as found in an academic minor and level of content integration across instructional formats. In this latter case, online instruction will offer a different type of resource to students, such as simulated environments, virtual tours, direct access to content experts distantly located, and prescribed tutoring. Face-to-face instruction in traditional courses will offer spontaneous student–faculty interaction, consideration of perspectives occurring in verbal and nonverbal dialogue, immediate mentoring, and formation of personal networks. Results of these diverse interactions may create opportunities to integrate content across the curriculum in different ways. Nevertheless, it will be important for students to gain equivalent skill sets of knowledge-based competencies. This reality generates a requirement that careful evaluation of student-centered outcomes directed by academic objectives be monitored throughout the curriculum to ensure a smooth flow of preparation regardless of the method of instruction, whether all online, all traditional, or a blended online–traditional approach.

Consistent with this theme is the decision regarding management of non-novice level courses and courses requiring acquisition and demonstration of knowledge application through direct care or motor skills. The practice-based component of clinical courses makes the approach to these offerings blended. Professionals with practice-based experience may expand their knowledge base with course content that is web-based combined with an actual clinical experience. Novice level learners may benefit more from face-to-face courses in which immediate demonstrations, return demonstrations, questions and examples can be given with new information and content either integrated with or running parallel to the clinical experience. Some online courses may be structured specifically in consideration of the level of learner similar to face-to-face course offerings, and registration may be limited by student experience. For example, a capstone leadership course may include the same content for registered nurses and generic baccalaureate nursing students but use different case based scenarios for demonstration and analysis.

Consideration should be given to the expected level of networking between students, faculty, and expert resources, as well as to the degree of direct faculty assessment that is embedded in the course and the level of interaction that will need to take place. This means that high level interactive mentorship built on the development of personal relationships as part of the learning and practice experience, such as a research experience, may not be appropriate as an online learning opportunity. Once the relationship is established, continuation of dialogue, discourse, and debate can occur over the web and may also be followed by web-enhanced environments. This type of support will distribute course materials and provide student access to resources on the Internet, as well as to communication between instructors and students.

CONCLUSION

In the future, online courses will make use of virtual environments in even more exciting ways. Holographic images may offer three-dimensional projections of individuals requiring treatment and presenting symptoms. Robotic labs permitting home-based interactivity may facilitate the practice of assessments and interventions. Improved color in digitized images and the ability to capture the sensation of touch in assessing tissue swelling and other physical symptoms will approximate more and more a real experience that can be used in conjunction with text-based and audiovisual communication venues. As technology grows, the challenge will be to ensure that students have the necessary skills to benefit fully from online offerings and that faculty are prepared to assist in the development and use of online education tools. The expertise of faculty will become evermore important, and the demand for direct access to these individuals will grow exponentially. The challenge will be for academic environments to recruit and retain these individuals in the face of proprietary industries.

■ LEARNING ACTIVITIES

- Using the web, identify three sites by which virtual physical assessment may be practiced. Evaluate the sites in consideration of their practical use and interactivity.
- Locate two online program offerings and determine the underlying pedagogical model. Identify the active learning components of the offering.
- Critique the balance of communication venues used in the two online program offerings and identify the most innovative pedagogical features.

REFERENCES

Anders, R., & Fechtner, D. (1992). *Universal design.* Brooklyn, NY: Pratt Institute Department of Industrial Design and Pratt Center for Advanced Design Research.

Anderson, T. (2004). Toward a theory of online learning. In T. Anderson & F. Elloumi (Eds.), *Theory and practice of online learning.* Retrieved February 18, 2005, from http://cde.athabascau.ca/online_book/ch2.html

Carnevale, D. (2002). Missed connections. *The Chronicle of Higher Education*, 49(8), A35–41.

Carnevale, D. (2003). Online spectrometry lab will let undergraduates try out costly equipment. *The Chronicle of Higher Education*, 49(35), A31.

Conrad, D. (2002). Deep in the hearts of learners: Insights into the nature of online community. *Journal of Distance Education, 17*(1), 1–19.

Dabbagh, N. (2004). Distance learning: Emerging pedagogical issues and learning designs. *The Quarterly Review of Distance Education, 5*(1), 37–49.

Facione, P. A. (1990). *Critical thinking: A statement of expert consensus for purposes of educational assessment and instruction.* Millbrae, CA: California Academic Press.

Maag, M. (2005). The potential use of "blogs" in nursing education. *CIN: Computers, Informatics, Nursing, 23*(1), 16–26.

Moore, M., & Kearsley, G. (2005). *Distance education: A systems view* (2nd ed.). Belmont, CA: Thomson Wadsworth.

Panettieri, J. C. (2004). Virtually perfect. *University Business*, 7(6), 40–45.

Shea, P., Pickett, A., & Pelz, W. (2003). A follow-up investigation of "teaching presence" in the suny learning network. *Journal of Asychronous Learning Networks*, 7(2), 61–80. Retrieved January 5, 2005, from http:/www.sloan-c.org/publications/jaln/v7n2/v7n2_shea.asp

Objectives

Upon completion of this chapter, the learner will be able to:

- Select appropriate teaching approaches to match course objectives and content.
- Transform on-site courses to online courses.
- Design learning resources and supplementary materials.
- Integrate various communication venues (e-mail, cyber chat rooms, discussion boards, and such) into online courses.
- Incorporate summative and formative evaluation into online courses.

Key Terms

Asynchronous Communication: Communication (written, drawn, or taped) between course participants (learners and faculty) that is separated by time intervals of varying duration.

Courseware: The computer program or package used to provide the course over the Internet.

Discussion Boards: Locations within an online course where learners can post questions and responses and discuss specific course topics or issues.

Discussion Threads: The organization of responses to individual items and/or postings into sequences based on the topic or initial posting.

Learning Activities: Assignments developed to facilitate learning rather than to evaluate performance in the course for grading purposes.

Synchronous Communication: Communication (written, drawn or videotaped) between course participants (learners and faculty) that occurs within the same time interval such that normal conversation is approximated.

Webquests: Structured learning activities that require that learners explore designated web sites and participate in online activities to facilitate learning.

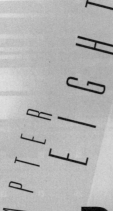

CHAPTER EIGHT

Design, Development, and Implementation of Individual Courses

■ NALINI JAIRATH

Chapter Outline

Issues related to development of online programs were addressed in detail in Chapter Seven. In contrast, this chapter focuses on issues related to the design, development, and implementation of individual online courses. Online courses exist in a variety of contexts. They may be part of programs that are totally online, or they may be integrated into programs that combine online and on-site education. Online courses may represent new courses or may represent transformation of existing courses that have previously been offered in other formats (Cuellar, 2002; Zucker & Asselin, 2003).

Although it is a challenge to develop and implement any course, online courses are especially challenging given the lack of coursework in pedagogy in most graduate programs in the health sciences. The development and implementation of online courses in all of these contexts require a basic understanding of principles of curriculum design and education instruction, which is beyond the scope of this chapter. Rather, this chapter focuses on the unique or specific considerations for online courses; it is written from the perspective of a faculty member tasked with developing and implementing an online course. As with many of the topics throughout this book, the literature relevant to the online environment is limited. Therefore, this chapter applies general concepts of course development and implementation to the online environment. In addition, this chapter draws heavily on the author's own experience with online courses. First, an overview of general considerations that affect online course development and implementation is presented. This is followed by a step-by-step planning guide for developing an online course.

GENERAL CONSIDERATIONS

When designing an online course, a period of reflection frequently precedes the actual processes of preparing a syllabus, selecting readings, organizing course content, structuring evaluation approaches, and actually implementing the course. During this period of reflection, faculty who are new to the online environment should consider the following:

- Courseware and software.
- Learner characteristics.
- Course objectives and course placement.
- Relationship between online learning and other forms of learning in the course.

Courseware and Software

Courseware is a generic term that refers to the software package or vehicle used to provide online courses. The courseware establishes the inherent skeleton and order for an online course by providing a template for course development, placement of course materials, and communication between course participants. For example, the courseware selected may separate out discussion items based on topic. This structure forces learners to decide where certain questions or ideas belong; in contrast, a different courseware program may combine all discussion into a long narrative thread, ensuring that all discussion content will be read. Some courseware may facilitate synchronous (i.e., real time) communication, while others may not. Blackboard (www.blackboard.com) and WebCT (www.webct.com) are examples of commercial software used to deliver courses. Courses may also be provided using currently free versions of sophisticated course management systems such as the Angel course management system (www.angellearning.com), programs from the Open Knowledge Initiative project (www.okiproject.org), or web sites created by course developers. Typically, when the course is part of a larger online program or when an institution offers several online courses, particular courseware is selected at the institutional level. Thus, one of the responsibilities of the course developer is to maximize the fit between the courseware and the way the course is conceptualized.

Courseware alone may be inadequate to meet the course objectives; additional software may be required. For example, online research courses may require that learners analyze data sets, or clinical courses may require that learners use software on a handheld computer (i.e., PDA). The course developer will need to consider how learners will be taught to use the software, whether the software must be purchased by learners on an individual basis or whether it can be accessed remotely and a site license for general use obtained. The course developer should also consider whether the software and courseware are compatible. If they are not compatible, teaching using software and courseware may occur in a parallel fashion, which requires more time and energy. To illustrate, if the learners in the research course do a group project, articulated software would allow output from data analysis to be imported into a file that can then be accessed by group members via a group home page. If the software does not articulate, the same output would have to be e-mailed to each member of the group. They would then open the output and examine it. Group members would either then e-mail each other about the output and possibly copy the course instructor. In contrast, if the software and courseware articulate, the output could be placed by one learner on the group home page. Group members could open the output while logged onto the course; and post messages that would be saved on the group home page. The faculty member could periodically monitor the group home page content.

Learner Characteristics

Learner characteristics are the second consideration in designing an online course. As with all courses, one should consider the general principles of adult learning (Knowles, 1990), the need to accommodate learning styles and preferences (Blackmoor, 2005; Kolb, 1984), maturity level, study habits, and preparation for academic coursework. However, additional characteristics that course faculty may need to consider include (a) motivation or rationale for enrolling in the specific online course, (b) capacity for self-directedness, and (c) computer and Internet skills and behaviors. A common pitfall by faculty is to assume that the learners are highly motivated and that they will avail themselves of the multiple learning opportunities available through online education. Thus, faculty may assume that learners are operating within the constructivist paradigm discussed in earlier chapters (Learning & Teaching Centre, 2001). In reality, learners may operate within an instructivist paradigm. They may take specific courses online for practical reasons. Learners in accelerated programs such as second degree or degree completion programs may carry a heavy course load such that an online course is selected because the learner believes that, out of all required courses, this subject can be most easily handled online.

Other learners may also view online education as an opportunity to insert coursework into busy professional and personal lives without recognizing that online education requires at least an equivalent amount of time and effort as traditional education.

The second characteristic that should be considered in designing an online course pertains to the learner's capacity for self-directedness. The capacity for self-directedness within an individual course may be influenced by the complexity of course material, its novelty, and learner knowledge and skills to be self-directed within the course. For example, in an online research course that the author taught to registered nurses in a BSN completion program, the novelty of the content and the learners' limited exposure to research resources impacted their ability to be self-directed. For effective teaching, the course should be planned to enhance learners' desire for self-direction and their ability to be self-directed over time. Faculty may develop learning activities to help learners become increasingly proficient in use of courseware. The complexity of these activities should increase over time and learners should receive rapid reinforcement for successful online behaviors.

The third characteristic that should be considered is the learner's degree of computer and Internet literacy and subsequent behavior (see Chapter Five for definitions). If it anticipated that learners will have limited literacy, it may be helpful to develop specific learning activities and orientation activities. For example, the faculty can devise web search exercises, exercises in which learners must download materials and exercises in which learners must use synchronous or asynchronous chat and group home pages. Behavior, or the degree to which the learner's literacy levels translate into specific behavior, such as checking e-mails, using Internet chat, and so on, must also be considered (Stokes, Cannavina, & Cannavina, 2004). In summation, when the faculty member understands the learner characteristics, the course can be designed to accommodate some of the learner limitations as well as to help learners develop necessary behaviors and skills for success.

Course Objectives and Course Placement

Ideally, the course objectives and the placement of a course within a program of study are key factors influencing the decisions made about the approach to teaching a specific course. Bloom's taxonomy (Bloom, Mesia, & Krathwohl, 1964) represents a practical approach to developing and analyzing course objectives as well as to linking objectives to the course format and course content. In this taxonomy, objectives may be considered in terms of the learning domain addressed (affective, knowledge, skills), as well as the competencies or expectation for learner performance upon course completion. These domains, which gained prominence over 50 years ago, continue to be used in online education, as evidenced in a relatively recent article by Woods and Ebersole (2003). Thus, objectives focused on description are lower level than those focused on analysis or synthesis of course content. In general, as the learner progresses through the academic program, the course objectives become more complex and will contain the higher level descriptors presented in Bloom's taxonomy. Furthermore, the more complex or higher level the objectives, the more important it is for the course format to offer opportunities to discuss and synthesize the course content. Thus, courses with higher level objectives are more likely to require a seminar or discussion component as opposed to a pure lecture format. Similarly, lecture formats are generally viewed less favorably for graduate level courses than for undergraduate courses. It follows, then, that an online course with higher level objectives such as the needs for synthesis and integration of information will require a different format than one with lower level objectives such as the need to describe or explore a phenomenon. Similarly, an online course that includes objectives pertaining to psychomotor skills will require a different approach than one focusing primarily on knowledge (i.e., cognitive objectives).

Course placement within the curriculum provides information about the other courses taken concurrently and indirect information about the capabilities of the learners who enroll. For example, if the credit load is high for the semester during which the course is taken, learner participation in the course may fluctuate as they balance the competing demands of multiple courses. Thus, it may be more important to use strategies to ensure consistent participation in the online course. If the online course occurs near the end of the program, the need to socialize learners to expected behaviors or to orient them to conventions for writing papers may be lessened. However, the need to ensure that learners can apply the content to their professional role may increase.

Ways in Which the Online Environment Can Enhance Learning

The last general consideration deals with identifying the potential benefits of the online environment for delivering course content and achieving course objectives. An online course allows the learner to gain repeated exposure to course material. Online courses allow a tiered approach to teaching. The course may be designed to allow learners to explore content matter in varying degrees of depth based on their interest. Online courses allow learners to use multiple methods of learning to master course content. For example, in online health assessment and skills training courses, the learner may have multiple opportunities to hear, see, and read about various skills. They may even have the opportunity to observe a skill being performed from several angles, sight lines, or viewing positions.

COURSE DESIGN AND DEVELOPMENT

Following the period of reflection, however brief, the faculty member begins the active period of course building. Ideally, the course should be built before implementation. No universal approach to developing the course exists, and the faculty member may engage in a process of fairly constant revision of the course as new issues emerge. In this section, common considerations are presented in a roughly sequential fashion.

A useful starting point for faculty assigned with developing an online course is to first consider the basic design of the course as it is envisioned or as it has historically been implemented; the term "design" refers to the overall organizational scheme or approach to course delivery. Courses in the health sciences have a variety of possible designs; common designs include lecture, seminar, assessment and skills laboratory, and clinical practica. Table 8.1 provides a working description of each of these designs, including the focus

Common Course Designs

TABLE 8.1	COURSE DESIGN	USUAL METHOD OF COURSE DELIVERY
	Lecture	Course content is delivered by the instructor in a lecture format supplemented by required readings; learners may receive lecture notes or copies of slides used in teaching at the instructor's discretion. The focus is on increasing knowledge.
	Seminar	Course content is acquired through classroom discussion directed by the instructor; learners and instructors may both present course content; and learners are required to have understood course readings. The focus is on increasing knowledge and ability to synthesize knowledge and understand its implications and on application in a broad sense.
	Assessment training and/or skills training	Essential course knowledge is provided through a combination of lecture, assigned readings, and audiovisual presentations. Basic mastery of skills is obtained through demonstration of techniques, practice during course times and in free time, followed by learner demonstration and teacher critique.
	Clinical practica	Essential content provided in didactic courses is applied in clinical settings. Course content is acquired through preparatory readings, clinical care experiences, and learner analysis of select aspects of the clinical experience. Most typically, learners synthesize prior knowledge and apply it to the current setting through learner written narratives (i.e., clinical logs or reports). An essential feature of this design is rapid instructor feedback followed by additional clinical experience through which skills are refined or consolidated.

and method of course delivery. All of these designs may be addressed using online course formats. In the case of clinical practica and courses with a laboratory component, the course may be administered online with learners accessing necessary clinical and laboratory resources at remote sites. In later sections, more specific information will be provided about how online courses using these designs may be planned.

A reasonable next step is to then decide whether the online course will follow the traditional design with accommodations for the online environment or whether it will use a different design. This involves consideration of the educational domains and the course objectives. For example, pathophysiology courses are typically developed to address cognitive skills; the broad goal is to increase the learner's understanding of various disease processes and the way in which certain conditions contribute to the physical course of a disease. However, within nursing and other health science programs, the learner is later expected to apply the material learned in a pathophysiology course to the process of providing clinical care. Traditionally, pathophysiology courses are delivered using a lecture format, with overheads or slides. If the faculty developing the online course decide to transfer the traditional format to the online course, then the online version could use taped lectures with commentary as a major way to deliver course content. Conversely, if the design is modified to reflect the way in which the course is integrated into the program, the online course could contain such content as three-dimensional images of the anatomic changes associated with the disease in question, as well as a streamed interview with an individual who suffers from the disease. This information, which could be easily provided online, could also enhance the quality of the traditional course.

Once the course objectives and overall design have been identified, the course must be built. This process involves having a visual image of the way the course will be presented online and then, structuring each element of the course in great detail. Online courses are less forgiving of poorly built courses than their traditional counterparts because of their greater transparency to the learner. Learners in online courses have the opportunity to repeatedly revisit material and thus can more easily detect its shortcomings. In addition, fine-tuning an online course during its implementation is harder because of delays in getting feedback from learners, faculty's limited ability to identify nonverbal cues indicating learner concerns or difficulty, and the reliance on information technology resources to make changes.

In online course building, it is helpful to address required resources and content structure.

Required Resources

Required course resources may include articles, videos, demonstration products, and so on. Identifying resources and their cost well in advance of the date a course is offered is essential to avoid potential delays. The faculty must also develop approaches to ensure that learners can access the required resources. First, strategies may need to be developed to help learners access course readings and other written material. Possible strategies include placing copies of course materials on electronic reserve via the academic institution's library system, scanning material into files placed on learner drives or on links accessed using courseware, preparing course packets available via mail or on-campus visits. All of these approaches take time to arrange. In addition, copyright permission must be obtained for protected material. Because online course material is not always treated as for single use by copyholders, copyright costs may be significant. Similar issues arise with use of videotapes or DVD material, and copyright costs may be even higher.

Second, tapes or DVDs must be digitized and converted into a format that can either be downloaded or streamed in real time over the Internet connection. The process of digitization, preparing material for downloading or streaming, typically requires the assistance of instructional technology personnel. Ideally, streaming is desirable because longer sequences can be viewed without delay or congestion on the Internet connection. However, streaming is only possible when the Internet connection has sufficient bandwidth. If bandwidth is inadequate, the images may appear jerky with sudden stops or mismatch between the audio and video portions. If streaming is not possible, or if the audiovisual material is lengthy, it may be necessary for the faculty member to divide the material into smaller sequences.

Finally, if demonstrations must be arranged in the course, time is required to assemble the necessary materials, arrange for the demonstration to be recorded and material to be digitized and then arranged for streaming from a web site. For example, in a physical assessment course, faculty must evaluate the benefits of using a commercial DVD or videotape to demonstrate the process of palpating the liver versus demonstrating the technique themselves. Similarly, if the course addresses X-ray interpretation, the faculty must decide how to present various X-rays online in a manner that approximates the way the X-rays appear in a face-to-face class.

Content Structure

Content structure refers to the way in which content is organized and communicated within the various sections of the course. The structuring of course content involves consideration of the (a) depth of presentation and exploration of course content, (b) method of delivery of specific course content, and (c) way in which access to course materials is timed.

Depth of Presentation

The content delivered in a course is determined by course objectives. However, online education allows learners to explore the course content to varying degrees depending on their time, interest, and expertise. A tiered or layered approach is possible with all learners exposed to basic course content but additional content may be helpful through access to optional links. This feature of online education is especially advantageous when courses are cross-registered at the undergraduate and graduate levels. It is also helpful when the class contains a variety of learners with different backgrounds. For example, the author developed and taught an online pain management course for nursing students. This course was cross-registered at the undergraduate and graduate levels. Graduate learners who took the course were expected to master the undergraduate level content plus additional content in recognition that they were preparing for advanced practice roles. Through receiving access to more in-depth content, they also had the opportunity to understand the pathophysiology of pain in greater depth and to explore pain in specific patient populations in greater detail. This approach was possible because of the online nature of the course. A similar approach allowed the course to meet the needs and interests of registered nurses in the baccalaureate completion program as well as those in the traditional undergraduate program. Although both groups of learners were undergraduates, the registered nurses were more interested in topics such as addiction, drug dependency, and drug-seeking behaviors than the less clinically experienced, traditional learners.

In developing a tiered approach, content mapping is invaluable. Content mapping involves clear delineation of the fundamental content that must be incorporated, based on topic area. In traditional courses, content mapping may be restricted to identifying the topics to be addressed in each class. In contrast, detailed content mapping is helpful for online courses because the teacher has limited ability to update or incorporate new content on an ad hoc basis once the course has been developed. Detailed content mapping also helps the teacher select online resources to enhance learning and accommodate diverse learning

Illustration of Content Mapping for Use of Narcotics for Cancer Pain Management

Tier 1: All Learners (Graduate and Undergraduate)

- Definition of narcotic
- Types of narcotics
- General benefits vs. drawbacks
- Side effects: addiction, respiratory depression, other side effects
- Use in cancer pain
  - Relationship to type and stage of disease
  - Dosing rates and regimen

Tier 2: Learners Interested in More In-Depth Information about Addiction

- Criteria for identifying addiction
- Addiction vs. dependence
- The relevance of addiction concerns in the terminally ill cancer patient
- Patient knowledge about addiction

Tier 3: Graduate Learners

- Legal considerations associated with prescribing narcotic agents
- Prescribing narcotic agents: impact of weight, disease process, and prior narcotic use upon dosing regimen
- Enhancement of pain management through combination therapy
- Alternatives to narcotic use

needs. Box 8.1 presents excerpts of a content map for an online module addressing narcotic use for pain management of cancer pain. In the example, content is tiered based on level of interest and learner status. Undergraduate learners are not required to explore the issues related to prescription of narcotic agents in as much detail.

Method of Content Delivery

Once course content has been mapped, it is helpful for the instructor to determine the most effective methods to present information. In online courses, content may be presented in video clips, slide shows or screen shots with voice-over narrations, hyperlinks to reputable online resources, through Webquests, lectures, and through other faculty structured learning activities.

Video clips are helpful for demonstrating skills or techniques. They are also helpful when topic areas are being introduced as a prelude to more in-depth exploration. For example, in an undergraduate research course, the author used video clips to orient the learners to new topics and to strengthen the learner's perceptions of a connection between the instructor and the learner. Videotaped lectures should be of short duration (15 minutes maximum) because of the passive nature of a lecture.

Slide shows or screen shots with voice-over narration are helpful when material will need to be reviewed more than once and when basic concepts need to be clearly identified. For example, when statistical analysis is being taught online, screen shots showing the exact way in which a test is computed are helpful.

Hyperlinks are helpful when excellent resources are available through the Internet, when learners need to become familiar with particular learning resources, when the opportunity exists for learners to explore topics in greater degrees of depth, or when courses are cross-registered at different levels (i.e., undergraduate and graduate level).

The *Webquest* represents a specific type of online learning activity in which the learner explores web resources in a guided manner. Webquests may be scenario-based with the learner directed to various sites in which knowledge about the topic is increased and through which attitudes are explored. Webquests may also provide learners with different learning opportunities to facilitate collaboration between learners and discussion of the topic. A Webquest may be developed for a specific online course or it may be in the public domain. Webquests are particularly helpful when attitudes are being addressed and the instructor is helping learners to use experiential learning. For example, in an undergraduate research course, the author used an existing Webquest called the Tuskegee Webquest (http://www.kn.pacbell.com/wired/BHM/tuskegee_quest.html) to help learners understand the way in which culture can influence what is viewed as ethically acceptable. Learners were directed to various source documents online to explore news events that occurred concurrently with the Tuskegee study. They then assumed various roles such as historian, sociologist, and scientist to explore how their role and societal content affected their perceptions.

Other faculty structured learning activities may also be used. These activities may occur within groups or individually. For example, in the author's online research course, learners were required to do a literature search using the Medline database to identify research regarding the nursing role in management of hyperlipidemia. They were then required to summarize their findings in one or two paragraphs.

Content Access

Content access includes sequencing and organization of content and control over learner ability to access content. All online courses need a structure; content may be structured by session, week, or module. The author has found structuring of modules most helpful in enhancing the flexibility of online courses. Structuring content by sessions or weeks alone is awkward because learners may use different timelines to access materials. The modular approach reinforces the main themes or progressive building of content or skills across a course. For example, when teaching a pain management course online, content on assessment of pain, principles of pharmacological management, nonpharmacologic management, and pain treatment in specific patient populations may be divided into conceptually discrete modules.

Once the approach to structuring content has been determined, the faculty member must make decisions about the sequencing of content. Content may be presented in a logical sequence or the sequence may be determined by individual learners. For example, in a traditional health assessment course, content may be organized according to body system with all learners learning about a particular body system at the same time. In contrast, with online courses, the same organizational approach may be used, but it is possible for learners to study body systems in a different order.

Next, decisions must be made about the timed release of content and the time frame within which learners must explore the content. Timed release of content ensures that learners stay engaged in the course throughout the semester. Thus, in a health assessment course, the teacher may decide not to release content about the renal system until after learners have completed coursework regarding the endocrine system. Timed release of content is pedagogically sound when content builds on prior content, when learners require time to master content, and when learning is enhanced through timely participation and discussion with other learners. Timed release avoids the phenomenon of learners who rush through all coursework at the start of the course. Conversely, timed closure of content avoids the phenomenon of learners who delay doing coursework until close to course completion.

COURSE IMPLEMENTATION

Ideally, the processes of course development and implementation should occur sequentially. In this section, factors that must be frequently considered during course implementation are addressed. Although these factors should also have been addressed during course development, they are frequently of greatest concern when the course is being offered, and they may necessitate rapid changes in the process of administering the course.

Learner Orientation

Learners need to be oriented to both the course and the process of online learning. Although it is desirable for orientation to online learning to precede orientation to the course, this option may not be available for small programs or when learners are enrolled in isolated continuing education courses. Course orientation should introduce the course, indicate how learners can access various portions of the course, and present basic information about the way in which the learner can seek assistance if necessary. The orientation should also address the affective component of online learning and promote development of a class sense of identity. Box 8.2 presents an excerpt from an announcement orienting learners to behavioral expectations and the general approach to course participation.

Technological and Other Usage Problems

The faculty should address the common technological problems a learner may encounter, indicate how learners may access assistance, and specify the turnaround time before a response can be generated and a solution expected. Learners should be familiarized with standard ways to troubleshoot when they have problems. Box 8.3 presents sample approaches to technological problem solving; the content was based on information embedded in one of the author's online courses. Such information may be embedded into a number of locations including the course announcements section, the virtual orientation for online courses, and discussion threads dealing with technological problems. Placing the information in several venues ensures that learners will not overlook the information.

Excerpt from an Announcement Orienting Learners to Course Expectations

 BOX 8.2

Getting Started: Course Expectations

Dear Learners:

Welcome to the web-based section of Course X. Some of you may have already taken web courses using Blackboard or WebCT; for others, this may be your first online experience. Based on my previous web experiences, I want to make a few comments, requests, and suggestions:

(a) Please recognize that this web-based section will require every bit as much work as the traditional sections of this course; in addition, you must be self-directed and use all learning opportunities provided in this course.

(b) Expect to spend the equivalent of at least 6 HOURS EVERY WEEK and much more time preparing for exams and assignments; this time is necessary to review the material for the week in the modules, to do the readings from the textbook, and to do the learning activities. This time is equivalent to that for learners in the traditional sections.

(c) The course is divided into modules, which have associated sessions. Thus, each module is comparable to several sessions in the traditional (i.e., non-web) sections. You are not expected to complete a module each week; rather your learning will be accelerated if you complete the portion of the module that corresponds to the session content for that week. The content for each session is indicated in the syllabus and in the course information section.

(d) For each module and within each session, learning activities have been identified. These activities are found as discussion threads in the discussion section of the course and are also included in the sides for each session. I do not assign grades for each learning assignment but rather view them as evidence of your participation in the course, an opportunity for you to test your understanding, and an indicator of your ability to master material. Thus you cannot fail a learning activity; however, if you do not participate or if your participation is minimal, late, or otherwise superficial, it is reflected in the homework assignment portion of your grade.

(e) Remember that Blackboard has several sections in which you navigate. The sections I use most are the discussion section under communication, announcements, and then the sections of course documents, assignments, and such. You should also check the archives for the synchronous chat sessions. These are important sources of information or clarification of information presented in modules. From time to time, I will refer you to especially useful chat sessions.

Sample Approach to Technological Problem Solving

Problem Solving Approaches and Contact Information for Various Online Problems Posted by Courseware Administrator

General Web-Based Course Concerns
E-mail online@xxx.xxx.edu (e.g., I can't hear the audio on video clips; the picture quality is jerky when I see video clips.)

Specific Course Content-Related Concerns
E-mail your instructor@xxx.xxxx.edu as indicated in the faculty area or check the discussion board for information (e.g., I will be traveling and have no access to Internet for one week; How many points is a particular assignment worth?)

Courseware Technical Concerns
E-mail coursewareadministrator@xxxxxx.xxx (e.g., How do I access archived sessions of the Virtual Chats? How do I indicate that I am responding to a particular comment in a discussion thread? My password is expired; what should I do?)

Browser or Internet Access Problems
Please contact your Internet service provider directly if you are experiencing slowness, being dropped from your connection, or difficulties with the browser.

Communication

Kaiser (2004) has emphasized the need to consider the concept of presence as an essential aspect of online communication. Three aspects of presence are important: connecting with students, being with them in a meaningful way, and being available. Although the concept of presence has not been fully explored in the relevant literature, it underscores the importance of carefully structuring communication between learners and faculty. Without structuring, online courses can deteriorate into a series of exchanges between individual learners and the instructor akin to a series of individual tutoring sessions. The number of exchanges can also multiply so rapidly that both instructor and learners avoid reading these exchanges. Therefore, the goal of communication is meaningful discussion of content in a way that is time efficient and also benefits the learning needs of individual learners and the class in aggregate. To appropriately structure communication, it is helpful to consider the following:

- The available methods of communication (i.e., e-mail, cyber chat rooms, discussion boards).
- The types of topics or issues for which communication is needed.
- Learner and faculty expectations.

Table 8.2 summarizes communication venues to address these specific issues along with specific approaches to address each of these topic areas. In general, for each topic, learners

General Categories of Learner–Faculty Communication and Recommended Communication Venues

TABLE 8.2	TOPIC OR ISSUE	COMMUNICATION APPROACH

	Orientation:
	  Technological
	    considerations
	  Fear and anxiety
	    about online
	    course
	  Need to connect
	    to other learners
	    and feel part of
	    a learning
	    community
		Frequently asked questions (FAQ) page
		Online course syllabus or outline
		Discussion thread or area focused on learner
		  introduction
		Early assignment of learners to course work and/or
		  study groups
		Learning activities that cement group working
		  relationships

	Technological and
	  other usage issues
		Virtual orientation
		FAQ page
		Dedicated e-mail addresses for technological help and
		  for individual course-related questions

	Performance issues	E-mail communication with individual learners Midterm and other periodic warnings Synchronous group chat and e-mail warning if learner participation in group project is inadequate
	Mastery of course content	Discussion threads or discussion boards Learning activity threads or learning activity boards

should know what they can expect, what behaviors are desired of them, and the time frame in which they can expect an answer to a specific question or concern.

Online communication for a course may occur via synchronous and asynchronous methods. Synchronous communication occurs with little or no interval between sending, receiving, and responding to messages. Most synchronous communication occurs in a designated virtual location such as a chat room or a virtual classroom. Usually synchronous communication does not extend beyond an hour. Unless the content of the synchronous chat is archived, this method does not benefit those not attending the chat.

Asynchronous communication occurs with an interval between posting a message and receiving a response. The content of communication is saved and accessible to all over a time interval. Asynchronous communication can accommodate the learning needs of both learners and faculty (Wiecha, Gramling, Joachim, & Vanderschmidt, 2003). It also facilitates more thoughtful communications because participants have time to think and reflect on their responses. It also provides an audit trail when faculty are examining learner participation. Asynchronous communication about a topic may extend for several days or weeks depending on the context. One limitation of asynchronous communication is that it may not build the same sense of cohesiveness as with synchronous communication.

The courseware may determine the exact way in which asynchronous communication venues are embedded in the course. Online courses may contain discussion boards or threads. They may also contain separate sections for learners to post responses to learning activities. The faculty may also use group home pages with specific group discussion threads. Using e-mails for learner to faculty communication should be limited because e-mails require individualized responses, which are usually not shared with the entire class. Therefore, they are time-consuming and have limited value for learning.

The use of the various communication methods is illustrated in an online, undergraduate research course that the author taught. In this course, synchronous communication was used to help learners review for exams. A virtual chat time in the virtual classroom was established approximately 1 week prior to exams. Learners were able to enter the virtual classroom and ask questions or discuss course content. They received immediate responses to their questions and more than one learner could participate in the discussion. The virtual chat was saved or archived; learners who did not attend the chat were able to access this archived material, and learners were referred to the archived virtual chat if they posted similar questions on course discussion threads or discussion boards.

Asynchronous communication was addressed via posted announcements, discussion threads, learning activities, and group home pages. The announcements were used to present general information about the course, to help learners determine how to respond to technological problems, and to provide course updates. Discussion threads were used to allow learners to discuss particular course topics. For example, a discussion thread regarding ethics in research might contain learner responses to content regarding ethical violations in the research process. Learning activities, a special type of discussion thread, helped learners to synthesize and apply course material. They also helped faculty to ensure that learners were learning appropriately. For example, one of the learning activities used in the course was to describe one research study pertinent to the learner's clinical practice. The articles identified and the learner descriptions allowed the learners to refine their skills in identifying pertinent literature and allowed the faculty to determine whether the learner could differentiate between clinical articles based on research, research studies, and literature reviews of the current research. Group home pages using asynchronous communication were used to allow learners in smaller groups within the class to communicate with each other about a group assignment in which learners analyzed research data and summarized their interpretation of the data. The faculty were able to answer questions posed by the group and to examine group process in preparing the assignments. Group members who did not participate in the group home page discussions or who did not respond to group member queries received a lower grade on the assignment.

Performance Evaluation

Most approaches to evaluation of learner performance approximate those used in traditional learning. In evaluating student performance, the faculty should address course participation and performance on assignments and examinations.

Course Participation

Learner participation should be periodically monitored when a course is being offered, and strategies to enhance participation and achievement of performance goals should be implemented. Learners who do not fully participate in the course or who do not meet their course obligations must receive clear indication in a timely manner that their behavior must improve. This information may be communicated via individual e-mails. If a group of learners is exhibiting similar behavior, the faculty may decide to address course expectations with the entire class. For example, an announcement may be posted reiterating class expectations or a discussion thread opened to explore why class communication and participation has decreased. Box 8.4, an excerpt from a course announcement, illustrates the way in which clear behavioral expectations of learners may be presented.

In evaluating participation, it is helpful to consider the frequency and nature of participation in course discussions and learning activities. When learner participation in the

Announcement Presenting Behavioral Expectations of Learners (excerpted from one of the author's courses)

BOX 8.4

Please note the following expectations:

(a) Technical problems or difficulties are **not** accepted as reasons for late submission of assignments, lack of participation in discussion threads, and so on.

(b) Learners are expected to log on **at least once a week** and participate in current discussion threads; their participation should show evidence that they have reviewed course content and that they are actively applying course concepts. Discussion threads may be closed **1 week after close of module.** Learners should differentiate between what is appropriate to post on discussion threads and what should be privately discussed with individual classmates or course faculty. **It is not necessary to send a duplicate copy of postings to Dr. Jairath.**

(c) All learners should be prepared to come on campus for the first and final exams. The exams will be held on the **Tuesday of the appropriate week and start promptly at 2 p.m.** Learners should make the necessary arrangements in their schedules now to take exams. The research critique exam may be taken online at a time mutually acceptable to Dr. Jairath and the learner.

(d) Group discussion pages will be established for learners to work on the computer assignment. If needed, Dr. Jairath may monitor these pages to determine the contribution of each learner to the group assignment. **A learner who does not actively work with the group and contribute the proportionate amount to the group project may receive a grade of zero for this assignment.** Thus in a group of three learners, each learner should complete approximately one third of the work.

If you have any questions, please post them in this discussion board area.

course becomes a concern, it may be helpful to use courseware to examine course utilization patterns. Commercial courseware may provide information about the number of hits or visits to the course, the parts of the course visited (i.e., discussion threads or discussion boards, learning modules, and such), and changes in the degree to which the learner visits certain sites or accesses course resources. Courseware may also provide reports on the total time spent on the course and may benchmark the learner utilization patterns against the average utilization patterns for the course.

Exams and Course Assignments

Exams, essays, and demonstrations or presentations are all feasible for evaluating learner performance in online courses. Although evaluation should be planned as part of course design and development, ensuring the security of evaluation approaches and rapidly addressing problems with online evaluation are major considerations when the course is implemented.

Security of Exams and Timed Assignments

Two concerns exist with respect to maintaining the security of exams and timed assignments. First, faculty must ensure that the actual learner takes the exam. Second, faculty may need to ensure that others do not gain access to the exam to prevent cheating and compromising of test bank items. In the traditional environment, security is maintained through the examination of learner identification, proctoring of exams, and retention of exam material. In the virtual environment, the instructor is not typically on-site to physically proctor exams and tests. Cheating may be facilitated if the security of exams is not assured. Sample cheating opportunities include the saving of screen shots of exam items, copying of exam items to files, and the use of substitutes or additional individuals to help the learner complete the exam.

These legitimate concerns may be addressed in several ways. Learners may be required to go to a test center or to have their exams proctored by a designated individual. Alternatively, eyeball cameras may be used so that the instructor can view the learner during the exam session. Each of these approaches has limitations. Test centers not affiliated with the academic program may have additional costs. Learner-selected proctors may not have legitimate credentials, and the process of establishing proctors is time-consuming. Instructor supervision of learners is cumbersome, blind spots for viewing may still exist, and the flexibility of online education is jeopardized.

Alternate approaches are to use existing capabilities in some courseware to randomly select test items from a test bank. Thus, each learner would take an individually generated exam such that cheating based on prior knowledge of exam questions is limited. This approach, however, will only work if a large test bank of items exists and if the reliability, validity, and discriminability of items are known and acceptable. Given these concerns, course faculty may elect to use alternate evaluation approaches. They may use take-home exams or exams with short answers, or they may elect to accept the inherent risk of online testing.

Technological Problems With Online Evaluation

Evaluation of learner performance may also be affected by technological barriers and difficulties. This is a great source of anxiety and stress to learners because most technological difficulties occur suddenly and without warning. For example, learners using various

Internet service providers may experience sudden loss of connectivity with no recourse to Internet until service is restored. Therefore, the course should have a clear policy and procedure to handle loss of service. It is helpful to specify (a) who should be notified of technological problems and the required time span for reporting, (b) how inability to complete an online exam or assignment will be handled, and (c) whether incomplete exams and/or assignments will be treated in the same manner as those that could not be started at all. In addition, during the course, it is helpful to have trial or test runs to ensure that the procedures for exam or assignment administration are operational and that learners understand the processes they should follow.

The second consideration involves assignments in which learners are required to give a presentation, demonstrate a clinical skill or procedure, or conduct an interview. In these circumstances, it is helpful to (a) consider the essential elements that a face-to-face approach provides, (b) determine whether alternate approaches are appropriate, and (c) if not appropriate, develop strategies to approximate a face-to-face approach in the virtual environment. For example, as an alternative to a group presentation, learners may prepare slideshows with voice-over narration. Alternately, they may film a presentation for streaming over broadband and then open a synchronous chat to address questions and comments. If sound is an important feature of the chat, learners may use microphones connected to their computers. When visual demonstration is necessary, it may be appropriate to require the learner to submit a CD, DVD, or videotape of the skill for faculty evaluation. Conversely, if real-time performance of a skill is required, the faculty may view the learner performing the skill if the learner's computer is connected to a handheld or eyeball camera. Finally, the faculty may use clinical proctors to evaluate learner performance at remote sites if a detailed evaluation guide is prepared.

CONCLUSION

The quality of online courses is enhanced when course development clearly precedes course implementation. The course development process is generally similar to that used for traditional courses. However, it is especially helpful to anticipate the communication issues that may arise and to develop course specific orientation approaches that incorporate unique aspects of online learning. A clear understanding of learner characteristics and motivation for enrolling in the online course may also help faculty structure the course to meet learners' needs and to harness the unique capabilities of online education.

■ LEARNING ACTIVITIES

- Conduct a web search to examine the various formats used in online courses. Compare and contrast the ways in which online courses with a clinical and nonclinical format are structured.
- Go to the web sites for various online courseware. Identify the strengths and weaknesses of courseware such as Blackboard (www.blackboard.com) and WebCT (www.webct.com) in terms of communication between course participants and presentation of course content.

- Do an Internet search to find an online presentation of Bloom's taxonomy. Examine the words used to describe objectives at different levels of complexity and difficulty. Next, find two course descriptions for online courses and examine the relationship between the format selected for presentation of course material and the objectives. Describe strategies that you would use to achieve greater congruence between course objectives and course format. To assist you with this learning activity, go to a web site such as http://faculty.washington.edu/krumme/guides/bloom.html, which describes the cognitive and affective psychomotor domains.
- Develop a brief Webquest to assist students preparing for faculty positions in the health sciences explore the constructivist and instructivist paradigms and their impact on the design of online courses. General approaches to Webquest development may be found at http://projects.edtech.sandi.net/staffdev/buildingblocks/p-index.htm and http://www.spa3.k12.sc.us/WebQuests.html.

REFERENCES

Bloom, B. S., Mesia, B. B., & Krathwohl, D. R. (1964). *Taxonomy of educational objectives: Vol 1. The affective domain.* New York: David McKay.

Bloom, B. S., Mesia, B. B., & Krathwohl, D. R. (1964). *Taxonomy of educational objectives: Vol 2. The cognitive domain.* New York: David McKay.

Blackmoor, J. *Pedagogy. Learning styles preference.* Retrieved September 5, 2005, from http://www.cyg.net/~jblackmo/diglib/styl-d.html

Cuellar, N. (2002). The transition from classroom to online teaching. *Nurs Forum, 37*(3), 5–13.

Kaiser, L. M. (2004). Presence in three interconnected contexts: Considerations for nursing education in the 21st century. *Nurs Leadersh Forum, 8*(4), 150–155.

Knowles, M. (1990). *The adult learner: A neglected species* (4th ed.). Houston, TX: Gulf Publishing.

Kolb, D. A. (1984). *Experiential learning.* Englewood Cliffs, NJ: Prentice Hall.

Learning and Teaching Centre. (2001). *Constructivism and instructivism.* Retrieved September 5, 2003, from http://www.worc.ac.uk/LTMain/LTC/StaffDev/Constructivism/

Stokes, C. W., Cannavina, C., & Cannavina, G. (2004). The state of readiness of learner health professionals for web-based learning environments. *Health Informatics Journal, 10*(3), 195–204.

Tuskegee Study Webquest. Retrieved September 5, 2005, from http://www.kn.pacbell.com/wired/BHM/tuskegee_quest.html

Wiecha, J. M., Gramling, R., Joachim, P., & Vanderschmidt, H. (2003). Collaborative e-learning using streaming video and asynchronous discussion boards to teach the cognitive foundation of medical interviewing: A case study. *J Med Internet Res, 5*(2), e13.

Woods, R. & Ebersole, S. (2003). Becoming a "Communal Architect" in the online classroom–integrating cognitive and affective learning for maximum effect in web-based learning. *Online Journal of Distance Learning Administration, 6*(1). Retrieved December 3, 2003 from http://www.westga.edu/%7Edistance/ojdla/spring61/woods61.htm

Zucker DM. Asselin M. (2003). Migrating to the Web: the transformation of a traditional RN to BS program. *Journal of Continuing Education in Nursing.* 34(2):86–89.

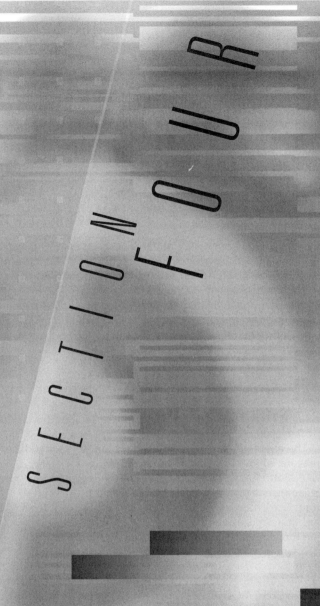

SECTION FOUR

Special Topics

Objectives

Upon completion of this chapter, the learner will be able to:

- Differentiate between evaluation of the instructor's performance and the course.
- Identify the general approach to evaluating online courses and instruction, including some basic principles of continuous quality improvement (CQI).
- Define the principle of triangulation and how it can be applied to the evaluation of online courses and instruction.
- Differentiate between the evaluation of online courses and instruction and face-to-face courses and instruction.
- Determine the rudiments of instrument construction.

Key Terms

Content Validity: A form of validity that determines if content is relevant to what is being measured.

Face Validity: The characteristic of an instrument that on casual observation appears to measure what it is intended to measure.

Formative Evaluation: An evaluation of processes in order to understand and improve them, and to better obtain the desired outcome.

Peer Evaluation: The process in which a fellow teacher observes a class and rates or makes comments about the instruction.

Reliability: The measure of whether a questionnaire or other instrument is obtaining consistent results.

Response Set: A form of bias in self-reported measures in which the pattern of responses of an individual is not related to the content of the questions.

Summative Evaluation: An evaluation that judges the effectiveness of a process, program, or intervention, emphasizing outcomes.

Test-retest Reliability: A form of reliability that measures stability over time.

Triangulation: The use of more than one data source or collection method to obtain different perspectives on a phenomenon or to compensate for biases in data sources or procedures.

Validity: The characteristic of an instrument that measures what it is intended to measure.

CHAPTER NINE

Evaluation of Online Education

■ MICHAEL MARANDA

Chapter Outline

Effective evaluation of courses and instruction is crucial to the implementation of a successful health services educational program. The advent of online courses is relatively new, and processes and procedures for evaluating them are just in the formative stage. Online pedagogy differs substantially from that used in traditional face-to-face courses. Techniques that are helpful in the classroom are often not applicable to the online environment. Online technology, however, through the use of interactive strategies, provides opportunities and approaches that are not available in the traditional face-to-face courses. As Diaz (1999) observes,

> Several forms of synchronous (real time) and asynchronous (delayed time) technology can provide communication between teacher and learner that is stimulating and that meets the needs of the learner. Information can be delivered in a variety of forms. Real-time "chat," "threaded" discussion areas, hypermedia such as audio, video and graphics, Shockwave, Virtual Reality Modeling Language (VRML), and Java applets are just some of the new and/or emerging technologies that promise to make the WWW compelling and interactive while delivering rich content. (p. 90)

The differences in the learning environment between traditional instruction and web-based instruction need to be addressed in any assessment plan of online instruction.

Although evaluating online courses and instruction provides some unique challenges and problems, the same evaluation and continuous quality improvement principles (CQI) that apply to evaluating face-to-face courses and instruction also apply to this mode of delivery. Furthermore, as in the traditional mode of delivery, there needs to be an integration of planning, assessment, and improvement activities for web-based courses. Course and instructional strategies need to be planned for web-based courses. Without assessment it is impossible to know if the plan was successfully implemented and if the implementation produced the desired results. If the assessment is not used to improve the course or to aid the instructor in improving his or her performance, then assessment is sterile. And, if there are no mechanisms or procedures to help instructors improve their instruction, then pointing out deficiencies may only frustrate them. Therefore, an integration of planning, assessment, and improvement activities for web-based courses is vital.

Before beginning this discussion, it is important to make a distinction that is seldom made but is necessary for effective evaluation: assessing the course and the instructor's performance are two analytically distinct issues that should not be confused. The need for this distinction is especially critical in health care fields such as nursing, in which students are required to learn a well-defined body of knowledge, and individual instructors often have little discretion in modifying a syllabus. In fairness to the instructor, it is necessary to distinguish between his or her execution of the course, which includes lectures, interaction with students, and the characteristics of the course, such as being built logically on previous coursework, having adequate library resources, and such. Furthermore, it is crucial for academic administrators to know what is working in the course and what is not, as well as the adequacy of support services such as laboratories or library resources as viewed by the students. For online courses, there are support services that are needed to facilitate online education that are not requirements for face-to-face courses. For example, technical support is crucial if students experience any technical problems connecting with the course. This chapter will discuss evaluating both online instruction and online courses.

Effective implementation of CQI produces a culture of improvement. A basic requirement for a culture of improvement is a supportive, nonthreatening environment where true communication can occur. CQI is nonputative in its orientation; information is gathered on products or on customers and is then examined. Strategies are then developed from these analyses to improve the production of the product or the services delivered. The results of those strategies that were implemented are then assessed. The process is iterative and done on a continuous basis. A CQI approach with course and faculty assessment works on the assumption that faculty would like to improve the course and their instruction and that they have the means to do so. This does not preclude using faculty evaluations of their instruction in their annual appraisal. Assessments of faculty's teaching should be used in the appraisal process to help faculty improve their pedagogical skills by identifying both strengths and weaknesses. Instructors need to know what they are doing that is working, as well as what needs improvement. The same is true for courses: Which modules are working? Are students using the interactive features? For the CQI process to be successful, it needs to be performed in a collegial and supportive manner, rather than as an authoritarian and coercive approach. In short, the emphasis needs to be on formative evaluation rather than summative evaluation.

The CQI approach starts before a new course is introduced. O'Neil, Fisher, and Newbold (2004) suggest a precourse evaluation for a new course. Before a course is implemented, external reviewers, without a stake in the course, should review the course for content and instructional design. Furthermore, the peer reviewer may continue to monitor the course during the first semester of its implementation. Champagne (2004), in contrast, argues that evaluation should be continuous throughout the course. Furthermore, he advocates that online courses take advantage of technology in order that the results of the evaluation be quickly reported to the instructors, so that they can improve the course as they are teaching it. He calls this approach embedded assessment.

TRIANGULATION

The principle of triangulation, put simply, is that multiple sources of information are better than a single source. Triangulation is a metaphor taken from geographic orientation; it takes at least two points of reference to locate an object in two-dimensional space. The two reference points and the object form a triangle. Further, triangulation is recognition that information may be biased or may represent only one viewpoint. Triangulation then may compensate for errors or biases that would come from using one source of information. Aerola (1999) and Appling, Naumann, and Berk (2001) recommend that multiple data sources should be used in constructing a comprehensive faculty evaluation system. In the case of evaluating an instructor's performance in a single course, the sources of information have been student assessments and peer or supervisor observation of the instructor. Students have the viewpoint of the consumer and the peer or supervisor has the viewpoint of a fellow professional. Another source of information is provided by the technology itself. Because the instructor's interaction online has been recorded, the instructor has the opportunity to analyze his or her interaction with the students.

When courses are examined independent of the instructor's performance, triangulation is also a useful approach. Student input again is needed, as well as input by faculty. A review of syllabi is usually performed by the faculty's curriculum committee, which may or may not include students as members. For online courses, it is critical to view the course itself. Because there are a variety of different approaches for delivering online content, it is important that these vehicles be assessed for appropriateness for the material presented, as well as their quality. In addition to student involvement in reviewing the course, it is also useful to have faculty from outside the school participate in the review. Because the students' time in the course environment can be tracked, it is possible to do an analysis of how much time students spent on various online activities. This may provide insight into which activities may be more useful to the students.

STUDENT RATINGS

The eminent evaluation expert Michael Scriven (1995) notes, "Student ratings add a valuable component to the range of input for the evaluation of teachers. Although many question the validity of such ratings, under certain conditions, results can and should be useful" (p. 1). Scriven cautions that the rating forms students use need to be crafted carefully, administered appropriately, and used appropriately. It is well accepted that teaching is a complex activity consisting of multiple dimensions and that evaluation of teachers should reflect this (Marsh & Roche, 1997). Students should be asked relevant questions about the instructor and the course that they can answer based on their observations. Furthermore, the results of these ratings should be used appropriately. For the results to be meaningful there needs to be a relevant comparison group. Furthermore, the emphasis should be on the pattern of responses to individual items rather than an average or global score. Neath (1996) cautions against using student ratings for summative evaluation.

L'Hommedieu, Menges, and Brinko (1990) conducted a meta-analysis on the research on student ratings and concluded that there is a persistent positive effect from student ratings. Mckeachie and Kaplan (1996) provide further support for the use of student ratings; they note that there is evidence that teachers use student ratings to improve their performance. Students are in a unique perspective for evaluating the instructor's performance and the course. As consumers of instruction, they view the course differently than instructors. Mckeachie and Kaplan also suggest that there is a benefit to student learning in filling out rating forms. If the form engages students, they are constrained to think about their educational experiences: What kinds of teaching and experiences contribute to their learning?

Student ratings are not without their detractors. There has been debate about whether or not student ratings correlate with the students' learning. Do students who learn more give higher ratings? This issue has not been explored in regard to web-based instruction. Regardless of whether student ratings correlate with students' learning, they can provide useful information on how the students view the instructor, on the instructor's behavior in an online environment, and what online activities the students found useful.

Student ratings are more important for web-based courses than the traditional face-to-face course. Web-based courses are more learner-centered than the traditional format. Mills, Fisher, and Stairs (2001) note that: "Feedback from students is invaluable in revising courses and operating procedures across the program" (p. 238). However, student-ratings for web-based courses pose challenges. First, any student rating questionnaire used for web-based course needs to take into consideration Internet pedagogy and the Internet environment. This includes the technical aspects of the students' online experience (Mills, Fisher, & Stairs, 2001). Course evaluation questionnaires used for traditional face-to-face instruction are usually inappropriate for online courses. These questionnaires need to be modified for web-based courses. Questions inappropriate for web courses need to be either eliminated or, where appropriate, reworded. For example, questions regarding the office or the instructor's availability after class need to be eliminated or modified to be relevant to the web environment. New questions that relate to online instruction need to be added such as "this instructor usually responds to e-mails within 2 business days".

For web-based courses, the student rating questionnaire needs to be online to provide easy access for students. A number of web survey packages are available that make the administration of student rating questionnaires relatively simple. The alternative is to use a package such as Access and construct your own web survey. This is usually labor intensive, and probably the cost in constructing it would more than pay for a web survey package. Web administration of course evaluations also need to be conducted in a way that assures the students that their responses are confidential and anonymous. Students need to believe that their responses will not affect their grade, in order for them to respond honestly. Scriven (1995) notes that when instructors collect their own student rating forms for their own classes, there is a potential source for error. Students may be reluctant to give their true responses if they think that the instructor can identify who gave the response. This view is supported by a recent study conducted by Fries and McNinch (2003). They administered two different versions of a student rating form to students in 24 undergraduate classes. The versions were identical except that one required a printed name and signature but guaranteed that the teacher would not see the names, while the other was anonymous. The analysis found that teachers received lower ratings on the unsigned forms for all evaluation items than on the signed forms. Furthermore, about 11% of forms requiring a signature were submitted unsigned. The authors suggest this means that some students are reluctant to give up their anonymity even if assurances of confidentiality are given.

Because it would be relatively easy to determine who submitted which answers from an online administration, the course evaluations need to be administered by someone other than the instructor. Because online administration is not an open process and students have no way of knowing who is administering the questionnaire and consequently who could learn of their responses, students need to be formally informed of the confidentiality and anonymity of their responses. If there are open-ended questions or a place for the student comments, the students should be informed that these comments will be shared with the instructor verbatim, if that is the policy of the school. The questionnaire also needs to be administered in a manner that prevents students from submitting more than one questionnaire for the same instructor–course combination.

Basic principles of questionnaire development apply to online student rating questionnaires. The introduction to the questionnaire needs to clearly state the purpose of the instrument, emphasize the importance of student feedback, and assure students of confidentiality and anonymity. In addition, the students need to be instructed to focus on usual or typical behavior of the instructor; they need to consider the whole of their experience in this course. Questions should not compare the instructor's performance to other instructors. Instead, it should focus on the instructor's behavior. Again, questions should clearly indicate that they are asking about typical or usual behavior.

One approach to developing questions is to have students agree or disagree with positive word statements about the instructor's behavior or aspects of the courser or ancillary services. Students can respond on a four-point Likert scale from "strongly disagree" to "strongly agree" with an option for the student to indicate either that this item is not applicable or that the student is not able to form an opinion (i.e., "do not know"). The forced choice format of the four-point scale constrains the students to make a judgment about the instructor's performance or the course (Appling, Naumann, & Berk, 2001). Furthermore, the four-point scale is easy for the students to understand; a six-point scale or greater would force the students to make finer distinctions than is warranted by the nature of what they are evaluating. Although it is usually recommended that a four-point Likert scale not be treated as interval data, it is useful for reporting purposes to report the results for individual questions as means. For more sophisticated approaches to developing question formats than the Likert scale, the reader is referred to an article by Schaeffer and Presser (2003), "The Science of Asking Questions."

Both faculty and student input should be sought for the construction of the student rating questionnaire. A collaborative process not only would more likely result in the construction of a better questionnaire, but also would promote student and faculty utilization of the questionnaire. Inspiration for questions can be derived from a variety of sources, including articles on Internet instructional techniques and teaching excellence, previously expressed concerns of students about online courses and instruction, and other schools' student rating forms.

In constructing individual questions, they should have high face validity; they should be straightforward and appear to be clearly relevant. Presumably, students will respond better to an instrument that is clearly relevant. Because the questionnaire is administered online, it may be relatively easy to allow a small number of questions that are unique to each course or to selective courses. Finally, it is good practice to provide students with an opportunity to include their comments about the course or the instructor. Students' comments may provide insights into issues with the course or the instruction or identify strengths about the instructors' performance or the course that were not specifically identified in the questionnaire.

Box 9.1 contains some sample questions designed specifically for online courses and instruction.

Any new instrument needs to be pilot-tested, and the results of the pilot test need to be reviewed before that instrument is used operationally. If the form is modified or altered, it needs to be pilot-tested and reviewed again before it is used operationally. Usually pilot tests are conducted with too few individuals to examine the psychometrics of an instrument. If the instrument is used for formative rather than summative purposes

Sample Questions for Online Courses and Instructors

Students can respond on a four-point Likert scale from "strongly disagree" to "strongly agree."

Evaluating the course:

- The use of multimedia (e.g., audio, video, graphics, and animations) was effective in conveying the course content.
- The online support resources (e-mail, discussion boards, FAQs, and virtual orientations) were helpful.
- Required electronic library resources were adequate.
- For this course, the use of technology usually enhanced my overall learning experience.
- For this course, the interactive online assignments usually were appropriately designed to assess my understanding of course content.

Evaluating the instructor:

- Faculty usually provided adequate individual attention to help meet course objectives.
- Typically faculty comments on assignments were helpful.
- Faculty usually responded to electronic communications (e-mail, discussion board postings) promptly.

and there is no overall score or scores for subscales, then it is probably not necessary to examine the psychometrics properties of the instrument. Under these circumstances, it is sufficient that the questions be clear, well worded, and relevant.

If the instrument will be used for a summative evaluation or it is deemed desirable to measure the instruments psychometric properties, then the appropriate measure of reliability is temporal stability, that is, test–retest reliability. The instrument should be given to the same group of students on two different occasions to see if they give the same responses on both occasions. Between administrations of the test, there should be no contact with the instructor. Because the questionnaire is measuring different aspects of the course or the instructor, measures of internal consistency (e.g., Cronbach's alpha) are inappropriate. The most appropriate measure of validity for these instruments is content validity. A group of faculty who have experience with online instruction but who were not involved with the construction of the instruments can examine the instruments to determine if they have content validity.

Two other concerns about online administration of student evaluations of instructors that need to be addressed are response rate and the timing of the administration of student ratings. There needs to be a sufficient proportion of students completing the rating form before conclusions can be drawn from the responses to the student ratings. A low response rate makes it impossible to draw valid conclusions from the ratings. Hence, students need to be encouraged to complete the online questionnaire. They need to be aware of the importance of completing the questionnaire. E-mail messages can be sent to the students reminding them to complete the questionnaire. Further, the questionnaire needs to be of reasonable length, easy to comprehend, and relevant to the course students are taking. If the evaluation instrument is too much of a burden to the students or appears irrelevant, compliance is likely to be low. With regard to the timing of administering the questionnaire, it should be administered after the students have had sufficient time to make a fair assessment of the instructor and the course and before the final examination to avoid the students reacting to their perceived performance on the final examination.

One final concern that plagues all self-report instruments is response set. In the case of student rating forms, two problems are likely to occur. The first is what appear to be random responses, where the student seems to respond randomly without reading the questions. The second is where the student gives the same response to all questions, possibly giving a global response to the instructor and course without taking into account variation from item to item. To minimize this problem, it is important to have clear directions that emphasize the importance of answering each question individually and the overall importance of student feedback. Other approaches include reversing the wording of some questions, so that some are worded positively and some are worded negatively, and including a dummy question (Porter, Blose, Valiga, Cumming, & Galloway, 2004; Suskie, 1996) that is clearly irrelevant. The following is an example of a dummy question that could be inserted: "This question is a placeholder; answer does not apply." If after reversing the wording of questions or the inclusion of a dummy question the pattern still persists, those questionnaires with the response set pattern can be eliminated from the analysis.

To interpret the results obtained from the student rating forms, it is useful to have an appropriate comparison group. Without a comparison based on some empirical data, it is difficult or impossible to interpret the scores; there needs to be some standard against which to compare. In the case of web-based courses, they should only be compared to other web-based courses. Furthermore, the comparison group should be composed, at minimum, of courses that are at the same academic level; undergraduate courses should be compared to undergraduate courses and graduate courses to other graduate courses. If there are sufficient courses, finer distinctions can be made. Once there is sufficient experience with student ratings for web-based courses, it is possible to develop benchmarks. Benchmarks should be set in consultation with the faculty. The purpose of benchmarks in a CQI context is to encourage improvement and to function as a guide in interpreting the results of the student ratings.

REVIEWING THE INTERACTION BETWEEN STUDENTS AND INSTRUCTORS

Online courses provide a unique opportunity to understand and document the interaction between the instructor and the student. Because much of the communication between the student and instructor is logged, the instructor has the opportunity to go back and review that interaction in order to gain insights that may improve his or her pedagogy (Jones & Harmon, 2002). The instructor can use appropriate qualitative analysis software to do a more formal analysis of the interaction or simply reread the material looking for areas of improvement. A simple rereading of the dialog between the instructor and students may provide the instructor with insights into his or her communication patterns with students. In addition, a more formal textual analysis of these data may also be of help in improving the course independent of the instructor. An analysis of the questions that are asked by students can identify areas of confusion that may be addressed by adding appropriate content to the online class materials.

PEER REVIEW

In commenting on the usefulness of peer review, Appling, Naumann, and Berk (2001) note that, "By providing an analysis of pedagogical content knowledge, course organization and structure, and effectiveness of teaching and evaluation strategies, this process adds a dimension to faculty evaluation that is not captured in student rating scales" (p. 251). To state it simply, advice from experienced teachers is usually useful in helping one to understand one's own teaching. A fellow teacher, either a peer or a supervisor, has insights into teaching that are not available to the typical student. To make the review more useful, a reviewer needs to identify both the strong and the weak points of the instructor's performance. In addition, the reviewer may be able to suggest ways to improve instruction. Although there is no physical classroom in which to observe, the reviewer can shadow the instructor online by observing the interaction between the instructor and the students. As stated above, web-based courses provide a unique opportunity to examine the interaction between the instructor and students that has already occurred. A reviewer can, with the instructor, review the interaction that reviewer has just shadowed to illustrate the reviewer's conclusions about the instructor's performance. They can also jointly review other interactions between the instructors and the students.

Peer review poses some challenges. It is generally believed that peer review is perceived by many faculty members as threatening. Certainly, if the review is conducted by a supervisor, such a department chair, the process may appear threatening to an instructor. As stated previously, this process has to be conducted in a collegial and nonthreatening manner. The results of the peer evaluation should be used for a formative rather than a summative evaluation. Thus, it is helpful to have faculty involved in the planning and the design of the peer review process to alleviate faculty concerns. To help the peer reviewers in their task and to ensure some degree of uniformity in the process, the peer reviewers should have some training and guidance in the procedure. Furthermore, the reviewers need a tool to help organize their observations. The tool may consist of topics or activities to observe and a place to record the observations. The tool may or may not have a rating scale for assessing specific activities. As stated previously, the reviewer needs to identify the positive aspects of the instructor's performance, as well as those aspects that need improvement. Although it is possible for the reviewer to observe the interaction between the instructor and student without either party being aware of it, it is not advisable because it can be viewed as more of a supervisory activity, rather than as a process of evaluation. Furthermore, it would violate the spirit of collegiality and undermine the trust that is the foundation of CQI. Brown and Ward-Griffin (1994) reviewed the literature on peer evaluation and concluded that its success depends on faculty involvement, short but objective methods, trained observers, constructive feedback for faculty, and open communication and trust.

CONCLUSION

Although evaluation of online courses and instruction poses some unique challenges and problems compared to the traditional delivery mode of instruction, the same basic principles of evaluation and CQI that apply to evaluating traditional courses and instruction also apply to this delivery mode. Because online pedagogy differs substantially from that used in traditional face-to-face courses, these differences need to be accounted for in developing instruments for evaluating online courses and instruction. Standards for online pedagogy need to form the basis of any systematic evaluation of online courses and instruction. There also needs to be an integration of planning, assessment, and improvement activities for web-based courses so that the results of the evaluations can be utilized more effectively.

Assessing the instructor's performance and the course are two analytically distinct issues that should not be confused. The need for this distinction is especially critical in health care fields, where students are required to learn a well-defined body of knowledge and where individual instructors often have little discretion in modifying a syllabus.

The principle of triangulation needs to be applied to the evaluation of online instruction and online courses. Multiple sources of information for online instruction include student assessments and peer review. Other sources of information are provided by the technology itself. Because the instructor's interaction online has been recorded, the instructor or a peer reviewer has the opportunity to analyze the instructor's interaction with the students. Also, the time students spend on various modules or online activities can be analyzed.

In implementing any evaluation process, the web environment needs to be taken into consideration. Standard evaluation approaches to evaluating courses and instruction need to be adapted to this environment. For example, student rating questionnaires need to be administered online rather than by a hard copy as is usually done in a traditional classroom.

For an evaluation system to be effective and useful, it needs to be a collaborative process, one in which administrators, instructors, and preferably students participate together. Furthermore, the emphasis needs to be placed on formative evaluation rather than summative evaluation. The evaluation process needs to be both an institutional and individual learning process wherein both the school and individual instructors learn to improve. To support this learning, the evaluation process needs to be conducted in a spirit of collegiality and support.

■ LEARNING ACTIVITIES

● Identify the differences between online instruction and the traditional mode of instruction that need to be accounted for in designing an evaluation.

● Develop some questions for a student rating questionnaire that would be appropriate for a web-based course but not a face-to-face course. What questions would apply to the instructor? What questions would apply to the course?

● Examine a log of student activity in a web-based course. How much time do they spend online? On what online activities do they spend the most time? Do you notice any pattern to the questions they ask the instructor?

REFERENCES

Appling, S. E., Naumann, P. L., & Berk, R. A. (2001). Using a faculty evaluation triad to achieve evidence-based teaching. *Nursing and Health Care Perspectives, 22*(5), 247–251.

Arreola, R. A. (1999). Issues in developing a faculty evaluation system. *American Journal of Occupational Therapy, 53*(1), 56–63.

Brown, B., & Ward-Griffin, C. (1994). The use of peer evaluation in promoting nursing faculty teaching effectiveness: A review of the literature. *Nurse Education Today, 14*(4), 299–305.

Champagne, M.V. (2004). Embedded assessment: An evaluation tool for the web-based learning environment. In T.M. Duffy & J. R. Kirkley (Eds.), *Learner-centered theory and practice in distance education: Cases from higher education* (pp. 283–294). Mahwah, NJ: Lawrence Erlbaum Publishers.

Diaz, D. P. (1999). CD/web hybrids: Delivering multimedia to the online learner. *Journal of Educational Multimedia and Hypermedia, 8*(1), 89–98.

Fries, C. J., & McNinch, R. J. (2003). Signed versus unsigned student evaluations of teaching: A comparison. *Teaching Sociology, 31*(3), 333–344.

Jones, M. G., & Harmon, S.W. (2002). What professors need to know about technology to assess on-line student learning. *New Directions for Teaching and Learning, 91*, 19–30.

L'Hommedieu, R., Menges, R. J., & Brinko, K. T. (1990). Methodological explanations for the modest effects of feedback from student ratings. *Journal of Educational Psychology, 82*(2), 232–241.

Marsh, H. W., & Roche, L. A. (1997). Making students' evaluations of teaching effectiveness effective: Critical issues of validity, bias, and utility. *American Psychologist, 52*, 1187–1197.

Mckeachie, W. J., & Kaplan, M. (1996). Persistent problems in evaluating college teaching. *American Association of Higher Education Bulletin, 48*(6), 5–8.

Mills, M. E., Fisher, C., & Stair N. (2001). Web-based courses: More than curriculum. *Nursing and Health Care Perspectives, 22*(5), 235–239.

Neath, I. (1996). How to improve your teaching evaluations without improving your teaching. *Psychological Reports, 78*(3), 1363–1372.

O'Neil, C. A., Fisher, C. A., & Newbold, S. K. (2004). *Developing an online course: Best practice for nurse educators.* New York: Springer.

Porter, J. D., Blose, G. L., Valiga, M. J., Cumming, T. L., & Galloway, R. N. (2004). *Controlling for random response behavior in a large multiple-institution student survey.* Paper presented at Association for Institutional Research's Annual Forum, Boston, MA.

Schaeffer, N. C., & Presser, S. (2003). The science of asking questions. *Annual Review of Sociology, 29*, 65–88.

Scriven, M. (1995). Student ratings offer useful input to teacher evaluations. *Practical Assessment, Research & Evaluation, 4*(7).

Suskie, L. A. (1996). *Questionnaire survey research: What works.* Tallahassee, FL: Associated for Institutional Research.

Objectives

Upon completion of this chapter, the learner will be able to:

- Incorporate key aspects of clinical simulation into educational planning for skill development and active learning.
- Differentiate between various methods of simulation important to clinical and laboratory course development and management.

Key Terms

Basic Simulator: Full-body simulator with installed human qualities, such as human sounds and childbirth.

Blended Simulation: Using multiple types of simulation to provide a comprehensive learning experience.

Computer Assisted Instruction (CAI): Passive and interactive programmable software.

Human Patient Simulator (HPS): Full-body simulator programmed to respond to affective and psychomotor changes.

Mannequin: Passive full-body mannequin that represents a lifespan and has exchangeable parts (i.e., wounds).

Standardized Patient (SP): Individual who is trained to portray patient scenarios.

Task Trainer: Part of a mannequin designed for a specific training function.

Web-based Simulation: Multimedia and interaction information accessed from around the world.

Virtual Reality: Complete simulated environment that includes audio, visual, tactile, hardware, electronics, and software.

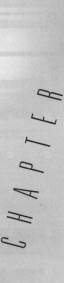

CHAPTER TEN

Clinical and Laboratory Course Development and Management

■ DEBRA SPUNT AND
DEBORAH SHPRITZ

Chapter Outline

Today more than ever, society insists that nurses and health care professionals be able to respond to the comprehensive needs of patients entrusted to their care. The students we graduate must be of the highest caliber and be able to meet the demands of a health care system under pressure. Health care educators face the challenge of designing effective programs to evaluate the clinical competence and validate the decision making skills of their students. Clinical simulation has been incorporated into the certification and licensure requirements for health care providers. Physician licensing exams as of June 2004 include: 10 hours of simulated patient encounters (United States Medical Licensing Examination, 2004); radiation technicians (American Registry of Radiologic Technologists, 2004); and nurse first assistants (Association of Operating Room Nurses, 2004) currently require competency assessment via clinical simulation.

Balancing academic and clinical education has been a challenge to educators based on the desire to produce health care professionals with a broad base of knowledge and clinical skills (Scherer & Graves, 2003). Didactic knowledge gained from simulations is retained longer than knowledge gained through lectures (Fuszard, 1995). The few studies measuring knowledge gained from simulations have found learning outcomes to be as good as those from traditional classroom learning, regardless of the type of simulation (CD-ROM, human patient simulators, catheter simulator) (Bruce, Bridges, & Holcomb, 2003; Engum & Jeffries, 2003; Jeffries, Woolf, & Linde, 2003; Jones, Cason, & Mancini, 2002). This type of educational program, however, is often the most difficult to design and maintain in a reliable, consistent, and standardized manner in the face of academic and clinical stressors, increased patient acuity, decreased length of stay, limited clinical experiences (agencies), and nursing and faculty shortage. Recent publications by the Institute of Medicine and the Agency for Healthcare Research and Quality emphasize the need to implement systems within health care education that ensure patient safety through performance standards. Institutions must continually improve their methodology of assessment of student skills by implementing practices and performance standards that will produce health care professionals equipped to meet the needs of an ever-changing health care environment and ensure patient safety. To prepare nurses for safer and more efficient practice environments while faced with the challenges described, nurse educators must explore innovative ways to teach nursing students about the real world of nursing in a cost-effective, efficient, and high quality manner. Providing students with limited clinical experience and immersing them in lecture content can impart technical knowledge, but this is inadequate to prepare them for the complexities of the workplace. Clinical simulation, combined with clinical experience and other teaching methods, is a powerful tool to prepare competent nurses for clinical nursing (Morton, 1996).

SKILL BUILDING AND THE USE OF CLINICAL SIMULATION

The nursing profession requires knowledge and skills to facilitate the timely and safe implementation of evidence-based practice, which addresses all aspects of health care. Nursing practice requires accurate application of technical skills and critical thinking. The Clinical Simulation Lab (CSL) provides an engaging, collaborative, hands-on, and student-centered learning experience. Simulations may be designed utilizing one or more simulation strategies, such as mannequins, task trainers, role-play, case study, games, computer software, and/or actors, which replicate clinical situations and the application of knowledge (Novotny, 2000). Simulation is an active learning process that fosters and encourages student inquiry and participation in an environment that is safe and nonthreatening, while providing realistic clinical simulation. This real-world setting facilitates transfer of skills practiced in the lab to the clinical setting and serves as an adjunct, not a substitution, to the clinical experience. Rather than isolating the technical skill performance, the lab provides for a learning experience that simulates comprehensive application of the skill in the clinical setting.

Procedural and problem-solving skills that focus on evidence-based practices are receiving increased attention because of their importance to patient care and the emphasis on rigorous competency standards being required by national organizations, credentialing bodies, and certification groups. The few studies evaluating skills using simulators or simulations have found that this method of teaching sometimes leads to quicker acquisition of the skill compared with conventional training methods (Ost, DeRosiers, Britt, Fein, Lesser, & Mehta, 2001). Simulation experiences also allow for the use of checklists as measures of skill competencies (Jones, et al., 2002). Overall, a simulation experience or laboratory is an ideal setting for students to develop psychomotor skills without any risk of inflicting harm to patients. To become comfortable and competent with technology usually requires repeated exposure to that technology, and this is easily accomplished in the simulated environment. The CSL provides an experiential learning component designed to maximize performance of selected skills and the application of concepts underlying those skills. The lab experience is integrated throughout the nursing curriculum and thus provides a connection between theory and the clinical component.

Time in the lab is facilitated to allow for adequate practice of skills and application to patient care scenarios. The student is provided the opportunity to apply knowledge from lectures and other resources in actual practice with the use of skills simulation (e.g., task trainers, computer assisted instruction, digitalized media), human patient simulators, virtual reality programs, and patient care scenarios. The goal is for the student to feel comfortable with the skill and confident in his or her ability to perform the skill accurately and appropriately in the clinical setting.

The CSL offers the student a learning experience that utilizes state of the art simulation equipment. The simulations enhance critical thinking, communication skills, collaboration, organization, and prioritization. This learning environment stimulates problem identification and problem solving. It fosters teamwork, collaboration, and leadership skills. It also provides exposure to clinical cases that may not otherwise be seen in the clinical setting but are nonetheless important for the student to master.

Role of the Instructor

Unlike in traditional didactic teaching models, the role of the instructor in simulation is that of facilitator. Rather than demonstration and return demonstration by the student, the instructor fosters success by modeling portions of a skill, facilitating the student's identification of principles previously learned, encouraging critical thinking, and identifying barriers to successful completion of a skill. An important part of this type of learning is based on planning on the part of the faculty. The selections of the simulator(s), scenario, and resources (i.e., web-based programs, multimedia) that will best meet the course objectives are essential to the success of the learning experience. A spectrum of simulators is available for faculty to utilize based on the student and course needs. Table 10.1 describes the spectrum of simulators that can be used individually or in combination to create an effective simulated learning experience. The instructor ensures adequate practice and testing time and is fully vested in the support and success of the student.

Role of the Student

Success in the simulation lab requires that the student come to lab prepared, self-directed, and motivated to actively engage in the learning experience. The student should openly interact with others, seek and share information, and not be afraid to make mistakes. Students learn best through active learning with assessment and prompt feedback (Tomey, 2003). Through simulation, learners are directly engaged in the activity and obtain immediate feedback and reinforcement of learning. Active learning activities can range from simple to complex. For example, a case scenario can be provided in which a surgical patient is restless and confused. Students are to assess and implement the most appropriate intervention and describe the rationale for the intervention. The human patient simulator (HPS) can provide more complex active learning strategies because the opportunity allows the student to assess a critical health incident (e.g., hypoxia, drug reaction) through the measurement of physiological parameters and communication with them, on-the-spot planning and appropriate nursing interventions, and real-time response by the HPS for realistic evaluation and further intervention (Nehring, Lashley, & Ellis, 2002). Case scenarios, real life-simulated clinical problems requiring assessment and decision-making skills, use of catheter simulators, role-playing with actors, and critiquing one's own or a peer's videotape of a selected skill performance are all methods faculty can use to promote active learning (Cioffi, 2001; Lee & Lamp, 2003; Morton, 1996; Nehring, et al., 2002; Vandrey & Whitman, 2001). Such active and interactive learning environments allow the student to apply didactic knowledge to clinical practice.

Role of Simulation

Simulation is a learning method that utilizes an artificial representation of real world events to achieve required performance goals. Simulations can be simplified versions or complex, but in any case, they must maintain enough realism to facilitate learning (Doyle, 2002). Simulation has been extensively and successfully used as a primary learning modality in the aviation industry, nuclear energy industry, and in military operations (Jha, Duncan, & Bates, 2001). It has also been used in the training and education of health care team members including paramedics, physical therapists, pharmacists, dentists, and physicians.

In the clinical simulation lab, various types of props are used to facilitate psychomotor skill attainment as well as application of critical thinking. Students practice on mannequins and task trainers and utilize computer programs to attain necessary skills.

Spectrum of Simulation

TABLE 10.1

TYPE	DEFINITION	EXAMPLES
Task trainer	Part of a mannequin designed for a specific function	IV arm, suture/drain model, Leopold palpation model
Mannequin	Passive full body mannequin that represents a lifespan and has exchangeable parts (i.e., wounds)	Resusci Annie, age-specific mannequins—baby to geriatric
Basic simulator	Full body simulator with installed human qualities (human sounds, childbirth)	Vital sim—Ann, Kid, Baby Noelle (birthing simulator)
Human Patient Simulator (HPS)	Full body simulator programmed to respond to affective and psychomotor changes	SimMan, METI
Computer Assisted Instruction (CAI)	Passive and interactive programmable software	Fetal monitoring, ABG interpretation
Virtual reality	Complete simulated environment that includes audio, visual, tactile, hardware, electronics, and software	IV simulator, robotics, data gloves, and helmets
Standardized patient (SP)	Individual who is trained to portray patient scenarios	Scenarios related to invasive and noninvasive physical examination, interview, patient education, and discharge planning
Web-based simulation	Multimedia and interaction information accessed from around the world	Access via hyperlinks to virtual clinical environments and information in action (time lapse demonstration of the development of a pressure sore)
Blended simulation	Use of multiple types of simulation to provide a comprehensive learning experience	SP—Interview Simulator—physical examination Simulator—intervention SP—education and discharge planning

Simulation is a learning method that utilizes an artificial representation of real-world events to achieve required performance goals. Simulations can be simplified versions or complex, but in any case, maintain enough realism to facilitate learning (Doyle, 2002). In addition to actual equipment used in the clinical setting, the lab is equipped with a human patient simulator (such as Laerdal's SimMan and METI), adult simulators, multi-sounds trainers, a birthing/newborn simulator, a pediatric simulator, and a virtual reality IV/phlebotomy simulator (such as Immersion Medical's CathSim).

Role of Human Patient Simulators

Human patient simulators (HPSs) are hands-on learning tools with computer-driven scenarios designed to replicate physiologic responses of patients experiencing and adapting to complex, multisystem dysfunction. In the clinical setting, health care team members are often faced with critically ill patients requiring expert, well-orchestrated interventions. HPSs such as Sim Man and METI allow for rehearsal of responses, team organization, problem identification, and problem solving. Students experience application of the nursing process in a simulated clinical setting and are allowed to interact with the HPS while addressing all physical, psychosocial, cultural, and spiritual needs. Scenarios are designed for individual as well as team intervention. The assignment of roles within the simulation can include that of the charge nurse, staff nurse, patient family, ancillary staff, doctor, or any other required role. With team intervention, the exercise includes all activities normally required in the coordination of patient care in the health care setting.

As with actual patients, frequent use of assessment techniques is crucial in planning nursing interventions. Heart, lung, and abdominal sounds can be auscultated with a stethoscope, as on real patients. Pulses can be palpated, blood pressure assessed, intravenous fluid started and infused, endotrachial tubes inserted, and other procedures as required per the prescribed scenario. A cardiac monitor displays a wide range of patient data, including EKG waveforms, pulse oximetry, and hemodynamics, which allows for assessment and response to critical events that may require further assessment, interventions, and collaboration with members of the health care team. These patient behaviors or cues are provided in response to the student's application of skills and knowledge to the simulated patient event. An important part of all simulation scenarios is the postsimulation debriefing. This time is used to analyze performance, critique the scenario, and brainstorm possible alternative actions. It is a time for positive feedback and a summary of events as well as providing for closure of the activity.

COMPUTERIZED SIMULATION

Simulation can be accomplished via multiple formats beyond the face-to-face laboratory. Technology in the form of computer assisted instruction (CAI) and the World Wide Web can be used by students as an interactive educational strategy. Computerized learning allows for use of multimedia and interactive simulations to critically analyze case studies in a safe environment that is rich in resources (O'Neil, Fisher, & Newbold, 2004).

Simulation-based materials allow the student to individualize the program based on learning preference and needs. Students have the opportunity to work independently or collaboratively as they utilize text information, audio (verbal information and recorded heart, breath, and bowel sounds), video (complete skill presentation, images from real clinical experiences such as surgery), graphic presentation of data (ABG results, vital signs over a 24-hour period), and motion images (visual demonstrations of renal perfusion through the kidney) to meet the course objectives (Zwirn, 1998).

Computerized, multimedia learning materials have been used to facilitate decision making in nursing when used with practicing nurses and students at the undergraduate and graduate levels. Case-based reasoning or clinical scenario reflects an educational strategy that uses coaching and the availability of technology-rich resources in the development of decision-making skills. This self-paced approach allows the learner to progress through the unstructured problem-based assignment from multiple perspectives and to gain insight into the clinical case and their own learning preferences (Kenny, 2002).

Clinical simulation, no matter which form it takes (simulators, standardized patient, computers, or the World Wide Web), is not a replacement but an enhancement of clinical in the real world with real patients. Simulation encourages and fosters independent learning. There is value in supporting students as they become self-directed lifelong learners applying knowledge to clinical decision making and practice.

STRUCTURING PRACTICA AND INTERNSHIPS

The increasing number of students in schools of nursing, coupled with the decreasing number of faculty available (AACN, 2003) to teach students in the traditional manner, has challenged faculty to find alternative approaches to clinical instruction. One method is the use of the clinical practicum using agency preceptors as clinical guides and role models for students. A preceptorship is a one-on-one contractual relationship between a student and a preceptor with a set time limit delineated at the beginning of the educational experience, while faculty retains overall responsibility for student performance and evaluation. Preceptorships in undergraduate nursing programs have flourished over the past decade (Bain, 1996; Haas, et al., 2002; Lengacher & Tittle, 1992; McCarty & Higgins, 2003; Trevitt, Grealish, & Reaby, 2001).

The preceptored clinical practicum can build students' confidence and self-esteem, increase the level of independent functioning, provide opportunities for role socialization, and provide opportunities for acquisition of competence and confidence in performing clinical skills, critical thinking and problem solving skills, and the application of theory to practice (DeYoung, 2003; Gaberson & Oermann, 1999; Oermann, 1996). In general, students' anxieties are reduced as they feel more comfortable demonstrating their knowledge and skills to *real* nurses rather than to faculty. Lambert and Lambert (2001) identify the roles of the preceptor as teacher–role model, workplace socializer, and coevaluator. In broader terms, the overall role of the preceptor is to bridge the gap between the reality of the workplace environment and the idealism of the academic environment.

Unfortunately, economic constraints and the shortage of nurses in the clinical agencies to serve as student preceptors challenge faculty even further to reconceptualize the clinical practicum. One way is to include an online learning component to the clinical experience. Through the use of an online learning environment, students can take advantage of clinical placements in sites outside of the immediate vicinity of the school of nursing and the clinical agencies where students are usually placed. Students can be encouraged to find their own clinical site and/or preceptor, which may be out of the immediate travel distance for faculty.

Using the online learning environment, faculty can post all course documents, including the syllabus, assignment guidelines, readings, clinical site information, pictures, and evaluation tools for easy access by all students at any time. Additionally, online guest lectures can be posted as an adjunct to the learning experience. Streaming video can also be used to review procedures or assessment techniques required for patient care. This is especially helpful for those students in remote sites and facilitates communication with faculty.

Because the preceptored experience does not usually allow students to prepare for clinical in the traditional manner, students often bring a number of references to the clinical sites, either in the form of personal digital assistants (PDAs) or a laptop computer. The technology enables students to access relevant drug references, drug calculation tools and calculators, general nursing resources, journal articles, and nursing textbooks. The laptop computer can also allow students to search the Internet for relevant resources on an as-needed basis that can then be shared with the preceptor and staff of the clinical unit.

Students can e-mail reflective logs to faculty on a daily basis with faculty providing feedback. Discussion boards can be used for threaded discussion (http://www.pitt.edu/~ciddeweb/FACULTY-DEVELOPMENT/FDS/threaded.html) and sharing experiences with faculty or their peers in other clinical sites. Students can also work online together on group projects and share the projects online with the clinical group.

Evaluating student performance cannot be delegated to the preceptor. Only faculty possess the skills and knowledge of the evaluation process for deciding student achievement of course objectives. Emphasizing this to the preceptor can considerably decrease a preceptor's anxiety. However, it is essential that faculty and preceptor communicate regularly. Because faculty seldom directly observe student performance in the clinical setting, the faculty rely on the preceptor's observations in order to judge the students' abilities or inabilities to accomplish clinical objectives. Tools describing student behaviors can be designed so that the preceptor can complete and submit them directly to faculty. If questions arise in assessing student behaviors, videotaping or videoconferencing could be used to allow faculty to evaluate actual student performance.

CONCLUSION

Technology is changing and will continue to change the way we teach and practice. Simulation by design focuses on student centered learning, which encompasses the student's ability to use technology to plan and provide safe and efficient patent care, no matter the clinical setting. The use of clinical simulation and preceptored clinical experiences help to ensure that students are able to meet the core competencies identified for all health care professionals by the Institute of Medicine (IOM). The 2003 IOM report *Health Professional Education: Bridge to Quality* (National Academies Press) identified the following competencies:

1. Patient centered care.
2. Interdisciplinary teams.
3. Evidence-based practice.
4. Quality improvement to practice and clinical environments.
5. Use of technology and informatics.

■ LEARNING ACTIVITIES

● Using a search engine, go online and access at least five physical assessment simulations such as heart and breath sounds.
● Compare the simulations for content and ease of use.

REFERENCES

American Association of Colleges of Nursing. (2003). *Thousands of students turned away from the nation's nursing schools despite sharp increase in enrollment.* Retrieved May 24, 2004, from http://www.aacn.nche.edu/Media/NewsReleases/enrl03.htm

American Registry of Radiologic Technologists. (2004). *Competency requirements for primary certification.* Retrieved August 24, 2004, from http://209.98.153.100/website.newsite/education/CompReqs.htm

Association of Operating Room Nurses. (2004). *AORN recommended educational standards for RN first assistant programs.* Retrieved July 28, 2004, from http://www.aorn.org/Practice/refaed.htm

Bain, L. (1996). Preceptorship: A review of the literature. *Journal of Advanced Nursing, 24*(1), 104–107.

Bruce, S., Bridges, E. J., & Holcomb, J. B. (2003). Preparing to respond: Joint trauma training center and USAF nursing warskills simulation laboratory. *Critical Care Nurse Clinics of North America, 15*(2), 149–152.

Cioffi, J. (2001). Clinical Simulations: Development and validation. *Nurse Education Today, 21*(6), 477–486.

DeYoung, S. (2003). *Teaching strategies for nurse educators.* Upper Saddle River, NJ: Prentice Hall.

Doyle, J. (2002). Simulation in medical education: Focus on anesthesiology. *MedEduc Online, 7*(16). Retrieved September 12, 2005, from http://www.med-ed-online.org.

Engum, S., & Jeffries, P. R. (2003). Intravenous catheter training system: Computer-based education vs. traditional learning methods. *The American Journal of Surgery, 186*(1), 67–74.

Fuszard, R. (1995). *Innovative teaching strategies in nursing* (2nd ed.). Gaithersburg, MD: Aspen Publishers.

Gaberson, K. B., & Oermann, M. H. (1999). *Clinical teaching strategies in nursing.* New York: Springer Publishing Company.

Haas, B. K., Deardorff, K. U., Klotz, L., Baker, B., Coleman, J., & DeWitt, A. (2002). Creating a collaborative partnership between academia and service. *Journal of Nursing Education, 41*(12), 518–523.

Institute of Medicine (2003). *Health professional education: Bridge to quality.* Washington, D.C. National Academies Press.

Jeffries, P., Woolf, P., & Linde, B. (2003). Technology-based vs. traditional instruction: A comparison of two methods for teaching the skill of performing a 12-lead ECG. *Nursing Education Perspective, 24*(2), 70–74.

Jha, A., Duncan, B., & Bates, D. (2001). Simulator based training and patient safety. In A. Markowitz (Ed.), *Making health care safer: A critical analysis of patient safety practices* (Agency for Healthcare Research and Quality Evidence Report/Technology Assessment, No. 43, Chap. 45, Publication No. 01-E058), Washington, D.C.: Author.

Jones, T., Cason, C., & Mancini, M. (2002). Evaluating nurse competency: Evidence of validity for a skills recredentialing program. *Journal of Professional Nursing, 18*(1), 22–28.

Kenny, A. (2002). Online learning: Enhancing nurse education? *Journal of Advanced Nursing, 38*(2), 127–135.

Lambert, V. A., & Lambert, C. E. (2001). Preceptorial experience. In A. J. Lowenstein & M. J. Bradshaw, (Eds.), *Fuszard's innovative teaching strategies in nursing* (3rd ed., pp. 242–250). Gaithersburg, MD: Aspen Publishers.

Lee, C., & Lamp, J. (2003). The use of humor and role-playing in reinforcing key concepts. *Nurse Educator, 28*(2), 61–62.

Lengacher, C. A., & Tittle, M. B. (1992). Critical care in a baccalaureate program. *Nursing Connections, 5*(1), 3–10.

McCarty, M., & Higgins, A. (2003). Moving to an all graduate profession: Preparing preceptors for their role. *Nurse Education Today, 23*(2), 89–95.

Morton, P. (1996). Using a critical care simulation laboratory to teach students. *Critical Care Nurse, 17*(6), 66–69.

Nehring, W., Lashley, F., & Ellis, W. (2002). Critical incident nursing management using human patient simulators. *Nursing Education Perspectives, 23*(3), 128–132.

Novotny, J. (2000). *Distance education in nursing.* New York: Springer Publishing Co., Inc.

Oermann, M. H. (1996). Research on teaching in the clinical setting. In K. R. Stevens (Ed.). *Review of research in nursing education: Vol. 7* (pp. 91–126). New York: NLN Press.

O'Neil, C., Fisher, C., & Newbold, S. (2004). *Developing an online course: Best practice for nurse educators.* New York: Springer Publishing Co., Inc.

Ost, D., DeRosiers, E., Britt, J., Fein, A., Lesser, M., & Mehta, A. (2001). Assessment of a bronchoscopy simulator. *American Journal of Respiratory Critical Care Medicine, 164*(12), 2248–2255.

Scherer, Y., & Graves, B. (2003). Acute care nurse practitioner education: Enhancing performance through the use of clinical simulation. *AACN Clinical Issues, 14*(3), 331–341.

Tomey, A. (2003). Learning with cases. *The Journal of Continuing Education in Nursing, 34*(1), 34–38.

Trevitt, C., Grealish, L., & Reaby, L. (2001). Students in transit: Using a self-directed preceptorship package to smooth the journey. *Journal of Nursing Education, 40*(5), 225–228.

United States Medical Licensing Examination. (2004). *Bulletin of information.* Retrieved July 12, 2004, from http://www.usmle.org/step2/Step2CS/Step2CS2004update.asp

University of Pittsburgh Faculty Development Service. Teaching with technology: Threaded discussion. Retrieved February 20, 2005, from http://www.pitt.edu/~ciddeweb/FACULTY-DEVELOPMENT/FDS/threaded.html

Vandrey, C., & Whitman, M. (2001). Simulator training for novice critical care nurses. *AJN, 101*(9), 24GG–24LL.

Zwirn, E. (1998). Media, multimedia, and computer-mediated learning. In D. Billings & J. Halstead (Eds.), *Teaching in nursing: A guide for faculty.* Philadelphia: W.B. Saunders Co.

Objectives

Upon completion of this chapter, the learner will be able to:

- Implement a strategic planning process for online continuing education using key indicator questions.
- Articulate design principles for online content development necessary to providing access to individuals, including those who are disabled.
- Design introductory information necessary for efficient participation of registrants to continuing education offered by webcast.
- Cite specific examples of future development challenges for online continuing education for national and international audiences.

Key Terms

Accessibility: The design of web-based content that makes it possible for disabled individuals to be reasonably accommodated.

Virtual Attendance: Participation in an online program offering that has no physical presence requirement.

Web Board: A secure, password-protected conferencing system.

Webcast: Video and audio recording of a live conference or program offering that is accessible via the Internet to registered participants as both a real-time or an archived event.

CHAPTER ELEVEN

Continuing Education Courses

■ MARY ETTA MILLS

Chapter Outline

apidly evolving technology, increasing clinical complexity, advances in treatment, and the emergence of new diseases are all factors contributing to the increased need for a strong emphasis on critical thinking and lifelong learning to retain and expand the competency of professional nurses. Further, the development of new clinical roles, the need for managerial and executive talent, the imperative to retain nurses in active practice over longer careers, and the desire by practicing nurses to move up the economic ladder lead to the demand for ongoing education to promote career mobility and development.

Online continuing education provides health care professionals with the means to increase their knowledge and skills, maintain currency with new information, and develop important networks with geographically dispersed colleagues. The nature of continuing education is that it is often short-term, specifically targeted on selected content, and not dependent on sequential building of themes over time. As a result, planning and implementation of these offerings vary to some extent from that of formal academic online courses.

The professional nurse as an adult learner is assumed to have a sophisticated knowledge of nursing, which is the foundation for the new content provided in continuing education presentations or faculty development programs. The American Nurses Association *Scope and Standards of Practice for Nursing Professional Development* (ANA, 2000) describe the adult learner as a participant in assessing, planning, implementing, and evaluating educational activities.

STRATEGIC PLANNING FOR ONLINE CONTINUING EDUCATION

Nursing continuing education activities should be planned and implemented in accordance with the criteria of an appropriate accrediting agency such as the American Nurses Credentialing Center's Commission on Accreditation. Strategic planning encompasses three key steps: (1) defining the method of delivery (e.g., online versus face-to-face); (2) market analysis of strengths, weaknesses, opportunity, and threats (SWOT) for developing and offering the proposed continuing education program; and (3) formulating recommendations for action implementation and timelines. The SWOT analysis outlined in Table 11.1 is central to the development of the plan. This analysis involves assessing the fit with the offering organization's mission, a detailed statement of the human, material, and financial resources needed to support the program, development of performance measurement outcomes including a competitive analysis, and evaluation of sustainability and marketability.

By its nature, online continuing education is intended to be short-term and able to stand alone in content. In establishing a strategic plan, the following questions can serve as a guide for planning:

Assessment: What content is desired or required by prospective participants? Who is currently offering programs in this content area? If other programs are being offered, to what extent are they successful and meeting market demand? How can the continuing education program be differentiated from competitor offerings?

SWOT Analysis in Strategic Planning

TABLE 11.1

ANALYTIC STEPS	ACTIVITIES
Assessment of consistency with mission	Define purpose and contribution to organizational goals.
Assessment of requirements for human, material, and financial resources	Develop budget; specify technologic assistance, equipment, supplies, and staff needed.
Determination of performance outcome measures	*For business:* State the number of offerings to be developed within specific timeframes, the expected number of participants per offering, and the income over expense to be achieved.
	For participants: Delineate the expected level of competency to be achieved by learners, and consumer satisfaction relative to program offering.
Analysis of competitive position	Identify other organizations offering similar programs, the source and number of participants, the cost of program production, the registration cost, the frequency of offerings, and the target market.
Evaluation of marketability	Assess the extent of unmet demand for specific continuing education offerings through focus groups, surveys, and test marketing of products.

Target audience: Who are the potential learners who would benefit from this content? What is the number of potential participants?

Outcomes: What is to be expected as a result of establishing online continuing education? For example, will this be a freestanding business unit or supplementary to a formal academic environment? Will offerings cover broad ranging content or service a niche market?

Time frame: When, and in what order, should programs be developed and offered?

Support: What materials and resources will be required to enable program success?

Content experts: Are appropriate faculty accessible to prepare the online educational activity in the required time frame and are they willing for their content to be made available on the web?

Operations: What technical and instructional capability must be in place to support the activity?

Finances: What funding resources are available to support start-up costs such as technical and instructional design support? What level of revenue will be required to achieve a return on investment?

Partnerships: What collaborative arrangements can be made to facilitate development opportunities?

Online continuing education offers an opportunity to respond to market needs through the creation of innovative short-term educational programs designed to assist professionals in building knowledge and skills. In order to promote new program offerings, there should be developed automatic broadcasts that are updated and sent to self-identified learners based on a learner profile identifying their specific interest areas. Using this method can greatly shorten the latency of distributing information about new offerings.

Administratively, the technical infrastructure must support the creation and management of learners' accounts, record learners' charges, receive online payments through secure web sites, and generate the appropriate certificate of completion and award of contact units after receipt of a completed evaluation.

AMERICANS WITH DISABILITIES CONSIDERATIONS

Online education presents some unique challenges for individuals who may have disabilities. Participants may have visual, hearing, and other types of disabilities that impact their ability to make use of this mode of education. This is especially important to consider in online continuing education because participants may not have had any formal experience with this modality or with the offering institution or its technology, making them less prepared to knowledgeably or technically interact with the online program. The geographic location of online participants may also be a factor in their ability to efficiently and effectively use the online continuing education offering because infrastructure support may be lacking in their location. Accessibility issues, as stated in the content accessibility guidelines (http://www.w3.org/TR/WCAG10), remind web content designers that users may:

- Not be able to see, hear, move, or process some types of information easily or at all.
- Have difficulty reading or comprehending text.
- Not have or be able to use a keyboard or mouse.
- Have a text-only screen, a small screen, or a slow Internet connection.
- Not fluently speak or understand the language in which the document is written.
- Be in a situation in which their eyes, ears, or hands are occupied or there is an interference.
- Have an early version of a browser, a different browser entirely, a voice browser, or a different operating system.

Accessibility requirements as guided by the Americans with Disabilities Act (1990), better known as ADA, delineates and protects the civil rights of people with disabilities and requires reasonable accommodations by public organizations to meet their needs. Public entities include any state or local government and any of its departments or agencies (such as community colleges). Although web-based offerings were not specifically addressed in the ADA, subsequent interpretations of the law address the Internet. ADA Title II deals with local and state (public) entities, whereas Section 504, Title 29, Chapter 16, Section 794 deals with similar issues on a federal level. Basically, the requirement indicates that electronic information produced by federally funded or conducted programs or activities needs to be put into a form accessible to students with disabilities.

Section 508 of the Federal Rehabilitation Act of 1973 was amended by the Workforce Investment Act of 1998 and went into full enforceable effect June 21, 2001. This section requires that electronic and information technology used by the federal government be accessible to people with disabilities, unless fulfilling this requirement imposes an undue burden. Section 508 addresses detail such as the need to provide "a text equivalent for every non-text element," "equivalent alternatives for any multimedia presentation that are synchronized with the presentation," and "pages designed to avoid causing the screen to flicker with a frequency greater than 2 Hz and lower than 55 Hz." This standard is intended to ensure that each individual can access content regardless of physical disability, such as those with vision impairment, and are protected from potential harm such as can be caused by the initiation of seizures due to rapid screen flicker.

DESIGN CONSIDERATIONS

Design decisions made at the outset of course development can serve to make online offerings more accessible to participants with a wide range of abilities and disabilities. Using a process referred to as universal design can be helpful in this regard. The Center for Universal Design at North Carolina State University (2002) has defined this process as "the design of products and environments to be usable by all people, to the greatest extent possible, without the need for adaptation or specialized design." These principles include the following characteristics:

- The design accommodates a wide range of individual preferences and abilities.
- The design communicates information regardless of user's sensory abilities.
- The design can be used efficiently.

There are some mechanisms that can be helpful in facilitating engagement by participants. Graphics and pictures can be verbally described or supported by text that can be accessed by participants in their desired formats, such as screen enlargement and videotapes or clips can be close captioned or verbally described. There are many web-based tools available to assist in the evaluation of accessibility (Table 11.2). These tools can provide an analysis of HTML web pages and a summary report regarding accessibility.

Design principles can also be derived from evaluation research by identifying measures that can be taken to promote effectiveness of learning, satisfaction, and practice outcomes, while reducing or eliminating barriers. One study (Curran, Hoekman, Gulliver, Landells, & Hatcher, 2000) reported increased effectiveness of learning resulting from the use of case-based online courses as opposed to text-based formats. This result was attributed to increased interactivity with case-based formats. In another study (Bennett, Casebeer, Kristofco, & Strasser, 2004), satisfaction with continuing education programs was found to increase when there were minimal technical barriers such as navigation requirements to access and interact with program content. This finding highlights the importance of including a virtual orientation to online continuing education for the participant who may be unfamiliar with the online mode of learning. Furthermore, programs should be structured to enable

Web Site HTML Accessibility Evaluation Tools

TABLE 11.2

TOOL	DEVELOPER	YEAR	FUNCTION	ACCESS
Bobby	CAST	1999	Automatic checks. Analyzes web pages for compatibility with browsers	http://www.cast.org/bobby/
Imagiware	Thomas Tongue & Imagiware Inc.	1997	Verifies links, spell checks, and performs some syntax checking	http://www.imagiware.com/RxHTML/index_noframes.html
Webmet	U.S. Government	1999	Four tools to test usability and accessibility as ease of navigation and readability	http://zing.ncsl.nist.gov/webmet/
Validator	Web Design Group	2000	Checks compliance with HTML standards	http://www.htmlhelp.com/tools/validator/

rapid transmission because this has been found to be as important to learner satisfaction as content (Chumley-Jones, Dobbie, & Alford, 2002), and links to other web sites and secondary data sources should be regularly reviewed and verified.

To enhance performance outcomes, the design of programs for continuing education must take into consideration that participants are not a captive audience and may choose to complete only selected portions of the content. As a result, the design should include modules with both technical and analytic skills. Each module of content within the program should have its own learning objectives, case studies, and data analysis examples related to real-life professional responsibilities, self-test activities, and glossary and should include online links to supplemental readings and resources (Farel, Pfau, Paliulis, & Umble, 2003).

CONTINUING EDUCATION VIA WEBCAST

Continuing education may utilize webcasting as a separate means of content delivery with the additional capability of real time participant dialogue via chat room support. Speakers must agree in advance, and in writing, that they are willing to be webcast and recorded for later postprogram access. Agreements should specify that the presenter consents to the recording of their presentation and the publicizing of any taped copies that are to be made available for purchase. If there is to be a waiver of any claims for liability on the part of the conference organizer, including for compensation in connection with recordings either at present or in the future, this information and release should also be specified in the agreement to be signed.

Program participants may access both live and archived portions of a program any time, anywhere, via the Internet. All registered participants should receive a letter confirming their registration for the program and indicating in which portion(s) of the program they have selected to participate via the webcast. Participants should be reminded that they will be able to access both live and archived portions of the program, such as a keynote address, selected lectures, and various breakout sessions via the Internet. Webcast details such as the schedule of topics, times, and speakers must be made available at a web site with a clear link, and participants should be provided with an online review of the technical requirements and set-up procedures for viewing a webcast.

Using a web board, live conferences may be accessed through a search engine by registered participants who are given an assigned username and password to this secure site. Participants are able to post questions for speakers preselected by the conference organizers for webcasting. They are also able to select lectures or breakout sessions in the designated conference for those speakers. Sessions are only live at the actual time of delivery, but can remain accessible for any period of time as decided by the offering institution. Frequently, archived content is made available for a period of 2 weeks to provide reasonable access.

Clear instructions should be provided regarding guidelines for asking questions of a speaker, setup procedures for access to the conference, and an opportunity to test audio and video access and quality. When the participant is ready to view a webcast, the participant should be directed to the web site to enter his or her user name and password and to select one of the dates and time slots of the desired webcast to be viewed. After clicking on the webcast hyperlink located within the session's description, the program will be accessed. Participants having questions for a speaker during a live presentation can post their questions online, and the online webcast coordinator can ask the questions verbally of the speaker so the participant can hear the answer.

The web board has the capability of tracking each participant's virtual attendance according to:

- First time logging in.
- Last time logging in.
- Total number of log ins.
- Total number of messages posted.

This mechanism assists in tracking both the number of participants and the geographic reach of the program.

PROGRAM EVALUATION CONSIDERATIONS

The evaluation of online continuing education programs may be difficult given that participants are not a captive audience and may choose not to complete an evaluation tool. Completion of an evaluation may be enhanced if a certificate of completion is not generated until the evaluation is submitted. Even so, registrants may not see a tangible benefit or credit for participating in the evaluation process. Because data from the evaluation survey are important to effectively reviewing program strengths and weaknesses toward continuous improvement, attention should be given to maximizing the return rate. The evaluation tool should be brief and take no more than 5 minutes to complete. Conforming to this length of time requires that only key information be collected and respondent burden reduced through the use of checkoff responses supported by a few open-ended questions. Although questions may include participant satisfaction with the quality of the online continuing education program content, structure, and technical considerations, the real outcome of program success is in its ability to assist users in obtaining and applying new or refreshed knowledge and skills. The evaluation should, therefore, include both fixed-choice and open-ended questions directly based on program learner objectives, such as acquisition of new skills and planned use of new skills.

Evaluation studies to date have largely focused on web-based learning as a mode of delivery, such as perceptions of online learning (Johnson, Posey, & Simmens, 2005), effectiveness of online versus on-site offerings (Lemaire & Green, 2003), and participant satisfaction (Atack & Rankin, 2002). Individual program evaluation has the opportunity to move evaluation into the specifics of impact on practice performance.

ISSUES RELATED TO ONLINE CONTINUING EDUCATION

Making continuing education offerings available to a broad audience, including international audiences, poses some issues that need to be carefully considered. Prominent among these issues are language and technical support. The language of the offering must be clearly stated with knowledge that participants may require additional time to read text or interpret verbal content. Technical support may not be available to the individual participant and the infrastructure supporting the participant's computer may be limited or problematic. For example, bandwidth or speed of transmission may make online content either nonaccessible or may drop the participant before access is fully accomplished. Depending on the geographic location of the individual, even electrical support may be sporadic. Clearly stating the technical support requirements and offering a trial test for participants can provide a means of self-assessment of program usability.

As the number of continuing education activities offered for audiences in the United States and abroad increases, it becomes apparent that some of the methods employed for the evaluation of domestic programs may not be appropriate for participants from countries outside the United States. For example, a demographic data questionnaire needs to include locations and positions that are not limited to the United States.

FUTURE CHALLENGES

As computer-based technology continues to advance, there will be opportunities to include innovative simulated environments that exceed the ability of today's skill simulations to increase knowledge and application of care techniques. One of the areas for development is a video-based clinical web learning environment that is interactive and personalized. These relatively open systems will be designed to deliver learning material via the Internet with the objective of improving learning effectiveness in clinical education. With advances in multimedia technology and digital libraries, it is feasible to develop more advanced multimedia-integrated, web-based learning systems that provide efficient means for storage, retrieval, delivery, and presentation of multimedia learning material. Multimedia involves technologies that combine several communication media such as text, graphics, video, animation, and sound. Clinical instruction video demonstrates detailed clinical procedures in a more explicit and clear manner than textual descriptions.

There are clinical education systems produced on CD-ROM that take advantage of clinical video (Prentice Hall, 2005), but they do not enable the tailoring of learning material to meet individual needs. The next stage of web-based learning will include the development of innovative approaches to content-based video indexing and retrieval. This will increase the usability of programs by making it possible for the user to retrieve specific content via keywords and to more effectively browse video. It will also allow for interactive questions and answers by having the system respond to ad hoc questions by searching multimedia content and retrieving appropriate information. In addition, individualized feedback to learners in real time based on personal learning histories and learning progress will facilitate the acquisition of new knowledge and skills.

New evaluation efforts will also need to be developed to directly assess the impact of continuing education activities on the quality of care participants provide in practice. Current methods rely heavily on methods of evaluating continuing education programs that are self-reported measures of knowledge acquisition and learner satisfaction. Given that the purpose of continuing education is to ensure professional competence and maintain standards and quality of patient care, evaluation methods will need to be developed that focus directly on the assessment of clinical outcomes, changes in practice, and improved patient care provided by those who participate in continuing education activities. This will require an expansion of evaluation efforts to include development and implementation of an impact or outcome evaluation component.

Evaluation of learning through testing and simulation exercises should be used to determine what teaching strategies should be used and what follow-up content should be recommended to learners based on their current level of knowledge. Design and development of an interactive model of continuing education in the future should also provide real time explanation, assessment, and feedback during tests and simulations to help learners identify errors and better understand concepts.

CONCLUSION

Online continuing education offers an opportunity to advance and enhance professional knowledge and skills for immediate application in health care environments. Preprogram planning is essential to determine the level of need and demand for program content as well as of resource requirements and financial viability of offerings. Necessary design considerations providing for accessibility, ease of use, and knowledge transfer must be built into programs with expert review and pretesting prior to implementation. Preparation of registrants through virtual orientation and direction as to technical requirements for program use is of key importance.

Continuous quality improvement through program evaluation is essential to building a constituency for programs subsequent to the first offering. Using evaluation and innovations in online techniques and resources such as interactive simulation and individual feedback will support advanced program development to assist in meeting the needs of future health care providers.

■ LEARNING ACTIVITIES

- Diagram a strategic planning model for online education using key concepts.
- Select one online continuing education offering or web site and conduct an accessibility evaluation.
- Locate two web-based skills simulations (such as heart sound assessment) and critically analyze usefulness to someone who is hearing disabled.

REFERENCES

American Nurses Association. (2000). *Scope and standards for practice for nursing professional development.* Silver Spring, MD: ANA Publishing Co.

Americans with Disabilities Act of 1990, Act 42 USC §12101, et seq.

Atack, L., & Rankin, J. (2002). A descriptive study of registered nurses' experiences with web-based learning. *Journal of Advanced Nursing, 40*(4), 457–465.

Bennett, N. L., Casebeer, L. L., Kristofco, R. E., & Strasser, S. M. (2004). Physicians' Internet information-seeking behaviors. *Journal of Continuing Education in the Health Professions, 24*(1), 31–38.

Center for Universal Design, North Carolina State University. (2002). Retrieved September 12, 2005, from http://www.design.ncsu.edu/cud/univ_design/ud.htm

Chumley-Jones, H. S., Dobbie, A., & Alford, C. L. (2002). Web-based learning: sound educational method or hype? A review of the evaluation literature. *Academic Medicine, 77*(Suppl. 10), S86–93.

Curran, V. R., Hoekman, T., Gulliver, W., Landells, I., & Hatcher, L. (2000). Web-based continuing medical education (II): Evaluation of computer-mediated continuing medical education. *Journal of Continuing Education in the Health Professions, 20*(2), 106–119.

Farel, A. M., Pfau, S. E., Paliulis, S. C., & Umble, K. E. (2003). Online analytic and technical training. *Journal of Public Health Management Practice, 9*(6), 513–521.

Federal Rehabilitation Act of 1973, Act XX USC §508.

Johnson, J., Posey, L., & Simmens, S. J. (2005). Faculty and student perceptions of web-based learning. *The American Journal for Nurse Practitioners, 9*(4), 9–18.

Lemaire, E., & Greene, G. (2003) A comparison between three electronic media and in-person learning for continuing education in physical rehabilitation. *Journal of Telemedicine Telecare, 9*(1), 17–22.

Prentice Hall Nursing. (2005). *Real Nursing Skills* [CD-ROM]. Upper Saddle River, NJ: Prentice Hall.

Web Content Accessibility Guidelines. (1999). Retrieved September 12, 2005, from http://www.w3.org/TR/WCAG10

Workforce Investment Act of 1998. Electronic and Information Technology Accessibility Standards. Section 508 (29 USC §794d).

Index

Page numbers followed by *f* indicate figures; *t,* tables; *b,* boxes.

A

Accessibility
  evaluation tools, 172*t*
  requirements, 170–171
Accreditation, 115
Action plan of existing programs, 25
Activities of web-based programs, 31
Adults, learning style needs of, 5–6
Americans with Disabilities Act (ADA), 65–66, 170–171
Assignments, timed, 137
Asynchronous communication, 134–135
Audiovisual learning strategy
  faculty-directed, 110–112
  student-directed, 112–113
Auditory communication, 109–110
Availability
  of continuing education to international audience, 174
  of developed courses, 94–95
  of resources, 7, 8*b*

B

Basic simulator, 159*t*
Behavioral expectations of learners, 136*b*
Benchmarks, 150
Benefit–cost ratio, 21
Blended simulation, 159*t*
Break-even analysis, 21–22

C

Capacity of web-based program, 30–33
Case-based logic tree scenarios, 112
Clinical and laboratory
  content and management, 115–116
  course development and management, 156–162
Clinical practicum, 161–162

Clinical simulation, 156–160
  HPS role in, 160
  instructor role in, 157–158
  simulation role in, 158, 160
  student role in, 158
Collaborative planning and decision making, 43
Commitment of existing programs, 23–24
Communication
  considered in course implementation, 133–135
  to faculty, 95
  faculty–student, frequency of, 97–98
Communication venues, 11*b,* 108–110, 134*t*
  auditory, 109–110
  kinesthetic, 110, 113–114
  text-based and audiovisual, 110–113
  visual, 109
  written, 113
Competency testing, 113–114
Computer-assisted instruction, 159*t*
Computerized simulation, 160–161
Computer literacy, 79, 124
Connectivity problems, 78
Constructivist approach, 12, 106–107
Content access, 130–131
Content delivery methods
  hyperlinks, 130
  slide shows, 129–130
  video clips, 129
  Webquests, 130
Content development, 46–49
Content mapping, 128–129
Content structure
  content access, 130–131
  depth of presentation, 128–129
  method of content delivery, 129–130
Content validity, 149